5000+ patients cured with

Zero Medicine/Money/Mortality

N.I.C.E

way to

Cure

COVID-19

A N.I.C.E initiative by
Dr. Biswaroop Roy Chowdhury

PRESENTED BY

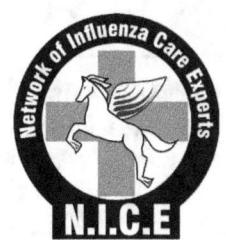

Network of Influenza Care Experts

BROUGHT TO YOU BY
Indo-Vietnam Medical Board

India Office:
C/o India Book of Records
B-121, 2nd Floor, Greenfields,
Faridabad -12003 (Haryana), India
Ph. :+91-9312286540

Vietnam Office:
C/o Vietnam Book of Records
148 Hong Ha Street
9 Award, Phu Nhuan District,
Ho Chi Minh City, Vietnam
- Hotline: (+84) 903710505

Malaysia Office:
C/o Bishwaroop International Healing & Research
PT 573, Lot 15077 Jalan Tuanku Munawir,
70000 Negeri Sembilan, Malaysia
Tel :+6012-2116089

Switzerland Office:
C/o Nigel Kingsley
Kraftwerkstr. 95, ch-5465, Mellikon, Switzerland
Tel : 0041 79 222 2323

FOLLOW ME

Facebook: https://www.facebook.com/drbrc.official/

Twitter: https://twitter.com/drbrcofficial

YouTube: http://www.youtube.com/c/DrBiswaroopRoyChowdhury

Instagram: https://www.instagram.com/dr.biswarooproychowdhury/

Telegram: https://t.me/drbiswarooproychowdhury

Email: biswaroop@biswaroop.com

Website: www.biswaroop.com

Published By:
Diamond Pocket Books
X-30, OKhla Industrial Area, New Delhi-110020
Tel.: 011-40712200
Email:sales@dpb.in   Website:www.diamondbook.in

N.I.C.E WAY TO CURE COVID-19 - DR. BISWAROOP ROY CHOWDHURY

A N.I.C.E. initiative by Dr. Biswaroop Roy Chowdhury

Our N.I.C.E. Consultants

1. Dr. K. B. Tumane *(Chest Specialist)*
2. Rehaas Habeeb *(Biochemist)*
3. Dr. Nilesh Patel *(MBBS Orthopedic Surgeon)*
4. Dr. Pallavi Patel *(MBBS DMRE)*
5. Dr. Hema Gupta *(Counseling Psychologist)*
6. Dr. L B Singh Chauhan *(Opthalmologist)*
7. Dr. Brij Bhushan Goel *(Naturopath)*
9. Dr. Vimal Kumar Modi *(MBBS, MD)*

N.I.C.E CORE TEAM

N.I.C.E Team Leader : Rachna Sharma

N.I.C.E Emergency Coordinator : Kalpna Bourai, Pratiksha Vats

N.I.C.E Coordinators : Emmanuel Job, Sameen Fatima, Shruti Sharma

24 hrs Frontline Officers : Harshita Ahuja, Alpana Tyagi, Riya Verma, Yogita Kashyap, Sonum Garg

Copy Editor : Dr. Shubha P. Wadhwa

Graphic Designer : Shankar Singh Koranga

OBSERVATIONAL STUDY
(All evidences in the book)

Our conclusion after successfully treating 5000 + ILI/Covid-19 patients with three step Flu diet:

1) The rate of transmission (R0) of SARS-CoV-2 is comparable to that of common cold.

2) The mortality rate of Covid-19 is comparable to that of seasonal Flu.

3) In the absence of social distancing, the retransmission rate and the chances of infecting a person (symptomatically and not diagnostically) is surprisingly less than 2 % .

4) Within the first 24 hours of three step Flu diet, the temperature comes to $\leq 100^0$ F for $\geq$ 90% of the patients.

5) Within the first 48 hours of the three step Flu diet, 60 % of the patients tested negative for Covid-19

6) Within 72 hours of the three step Flu diet,
   (i) All symptoms were resolved for approximately 80% of the patients.
   (ii) 75 % of the patients tested negative for Covid-19

7) With the three step Flu diet for 3 days followed by D.I.P. Diet:
   • 95 % of the patients recovered within 7 days
   • 100 % of the patients recovered within 14 days

8) It is possible to successfully treat severely ill ILI/Covid-19 patients in home setting with zero medicines/without oxygen cylinders or external respiratory support. Severely ill means:
   • Temperature $\geq 104^0$F
   • $SpO_2 \leq 75$ %
   • Severe Pneumonia
   • Acute Respiratory Distress Syndrome

9) For more than 95% of the patients and their family members, the panic situation is not due to symptoms/physical discomfort rather it is due to the Covid-19 phobia and fear psychosis.

DEDICATION

Dedicated to my angel daughter Ivy,

loving wife Neerja

&

caring parents

Shri Bikash Roy Chowdhury

Shrimati Lila Roy Chowdhury

CONTENTS

SECTION - I

SECTION - II

SECTION-I

CHAPTER-1

Solving the Mystery of Covid-19

I have a rare privilege of treating and curing more than 5000 patients that too, at the peak of the pandemic between June 5, 2020 and July 14, 2020. All this has been possible with the help of my network of more than 200 Influenza Experts spread all across the country (and few outside the country also).

We achieved cent per cent cure with zero medication and zero per cent mortality, with more than 80% of the patients, who could resolve their symptoms in 72 hours of following the three day Flu diet (details of which are given in the chapters that follow) and 75% of the patients (among those who went for second RT-PCR test for SARS-CoV-2) tested negative for SARS-CoV-2.

The above results may be baffling and may look manipulated and over exaggerated for conventional doctors with a mindset of treating Influenza/Covid-19 patients with the medicine protocol set by WHO, where they are used to see about 3-4% mortality with average hospital discharge rate of 14 days, but for me, the mystery was something else.

Out of the 5000 + patients with the classical Influenza like illness (ILI) symptoms as defined by CDC, about 1000 patients came to us with SARS-CoV-2 positive test report through RT-PCR, and the rest came to us without going for RT-PCR test for Covid-19. This means, out of 5000 ILI patients, 1000 were Covid-19 patients and rest 4000 were non Covid-19 ILI patients.

If we go by the guidelines of issuing death certificates released by ICMR[1](Indian Council of Medical Research), if any person dies with the classical symptoms of ILI, then the cause of death should be mentioned as Covid-19 even if the RT-PCR test for SARS-CoV-2 is negative before or after the death. This means, ICMR believes that 100% of ILI patients have a single causative agent and that should be SARS-CoV-2, although this theory of ICMR does not have any evidence in the medical literature.

Going by the guidelines of "How to Report in Death Certificates" by ICMR, technically, I should say that in the last 40 days, we have cured 5000+ Covid-19 patients. However, the causative agent of the symptoms of Flu or ILI can be among more than 200 viruses as identified till date and also, it could be other pathogens including bacteria, fungi and even non-parasite cause including side effects of the drugs etc.

The mystery for me while treating these 5000+ patients was that I could not find any particular symptom among the ILI patients with Covid-19 positive status which is unique to them (1000 patients with positive RT-PCR report) and can be distinguishable from the rest of 4000 patients (surely many out of them might be having causative agent other than SARS-CoV-2).

My First Conclusion...

Symptomatically, Covid-19 patients are identical to other ILI patients with no unique sign or pattern of recovery.

To unfold the mystery rather to solve the puzzle called Covid-19, I will take you to the first week of January 2020 (around 4-7 January) with the headline in most of the newspapers across the world "Cause of Wuhan's mysterious Pneumonia cases still unknown, Chinese officials say",[2] which even WHO acknowledged on January 5, 2020 on their website[3].

As per WHO, on January 3, 2020[4], a total of 44 patients with

Pneumonia of unknown etiology were reported by the national authorities of China.

Knowing that each year more than 2.5 million[5] people die of Pneumonia and around 450 million population, who suffers from Pneumonia or ILI, the intriguing question is how the health authorities distinguish those reported 44 patients as Pneumonia with unknown etiology. Let's have a look at the following facts:
1) In more than 60% of the ILI, no virus could be detected.[6]
2) In more than 20% of Pneumonia, no causative agent could be detected. [7]

My Argument

1. All across the world including your neighbourhood, for every ten patients with ILI (symptomatically) at least six will not be detected with any of the virus known for ILI.
2. For every ten patients with Pneumonia, at least two will not be detected with any unknown causative agent.

Meaning thereby that more than 60% patients with ILI can be called as ILI patients with unknown etiology (cause)

And

20% of Pneumonia patients with unknown etiology

Or

20% of them can be called as mysterious Pneumonia.

Here, I must remind you that symptomatically, the Covid-19 patients do not show any unique characteristics or sign or pattern that is distinguishable from other ILI/Pneumonia patients and also it is literally not possible to rule out all the known causes of Pneumonia as there are thousands of causative agents which may lead to Pneumonia. Diagnostically, the best tool available to science is PCR test (which is known as gold standard) but with high false positive meaning that when PCR test will be conducted for more than 200 viruses known to humans, to be the causative agent of ILI/ Pneumonia, statistically (on an average) it will show positive for at least two of the 200 viruses, even in the absence of any of the 200 viruses, since the specificity of PCR-test, by design cannot be more than 99%,[8] which translates to showing two viruses as a causative agent, even if none of them may be present.

Now, virtually there are no means to know, whether the test positive is a TRUE positive or FALSE positive.

Conclusively, the positive result (even though it is FALSE positive) could be accepted as a causative agent of the ILI for a particular patient.

Hence, the question is what was the basis of deciding that the causative agent of Pneumonia among the 44 patients is of unknown etiology. I tried to refer to the WHO website at the link (see the box below) but the matter does not exist.

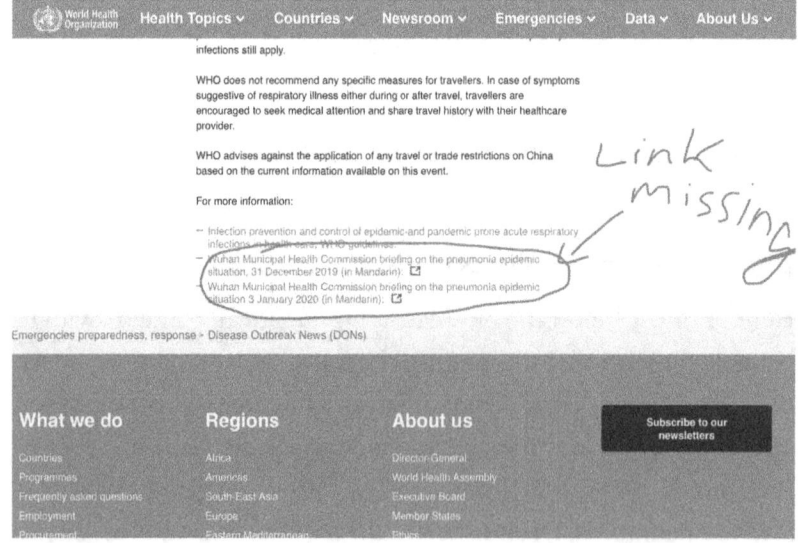

Since WHO and China health authorities have not given any data or evidence or study to prove, how can they rule out the possibility of all known causes for Pneumonia and also how they came to the conclusion that SARS-CoV-2 may be the causative agent of Pneumonia among those 44 patients, and even if it is the causative agent, it may not be a new virus to the human being, rather may be one of the causative agents of Pneumonia among those 20% patients, for whom causative agent could not be detected earlier.

In simple language, SARS-CoV-2 may have been causing ILI/ Pneumonia since long, but it is now we devised a method to detect the virus.

My Conclusion

Based on my experience of treating 5000+ patients and also with the above evidence, we can conclude that SARS-CoV-2 is not a new virus, with no unique illness/symptom, specially when WHO or China has not given any evidence to prove it to be a new virus.

Hence announcing Pandemic is technically wrong as by definition[9] Pandemic means worldwide spread of a new disease. If we talk of India, even the Epidemic Act 1897, as implemented by the Government of India is unconstitutional and unwarranted since by WHO definition,[10] epidemic means occurrence of an illness clearly in excess of normal expectancy. For India, the average number of deaths due to Pneumonia is 1.5 lakh per year and also the death due to Covid-19 as on July 13, 2020 is 22, 000 which may not be true Covid deaths, rather deaths with SARS-CoV-2 due to experimental medical procedures and co-morbid conditions (as explained in the later chapters).

We must remind ourselves that the basis of lockdown and social distancing with the announcement of Pandemic and implementation of Epidemic Act was the following prediction[11] by WHO in the month of March 2020.

Prediction no1
Prediction for the world

If no lockdown or social distancing or other preventive measures are taken then nearly 4 crore people will be killed worldwide and if all the prevention and lockdown measures are followed even then 2 crore people will die worldwide in the next few months.

Prediction no 2
Prediction for India

If no lockdown or social distancing or other preventive measures are taken, then up to 60,96,359 people will die and if all the WHO guidelines of lockdown or social distancing are followed then about 23,75,803 people will be killed due to Covid-19 in the next few months.

Now with serology survey by ICMR, it is established that the Case Fatality Rate (CFR) of Covid-19 is 0.08%,[12] which is lower than the seasonal Flu and the rate of transmission (RO) is 1.15[13] which is less than the common cold, meaning thereby Covid-19 is neither deadly nor infectious as has been predicted and projected.

Fortunately, with a very low CFR and RO, the death worldwide and also in India, is nowhere near to the WHO prediction.

Hence to normalize everything around, we just need to erase three words from our lives:

It is not a MYSTERIOUS virus

NO EPIDEMIC

NO PANDEMIC

Through repeated hammering and through media and phone caller tune, you are made to believe that it is a mysterious deadly virus causing high casualty, but with no supportive evidence.

References :

To access the references related to this chapter, go to the link : www.biswaroop.com/nicebook

CHAPTER-2

Why so many Corona deaths?
Answer in Three Steps
How to Cure Covid-19?

(Based on the lecture delivered on June 5, 2020 at the launch of N.I.C.E.)

How can one become a warrior? For this, I was making a framework for the last two months named as N.I.C.E. (Network of Influenza Care Experts) and it was launched on June 5, 2020 at 5 pm on the occasion of World Environment day. It is a network of trained people spread across the entire country and after the launch, if there is a symptom of ILI/Flu (I don't call it Corona), due care will be provided to that person absolutely free of cost. Till the person recovers completely, he would be under our support system.

Let us first talk about the entire game. Everyone is surprised as to why so many deaths are occurring? Why so many people are dying in Brazil, Spain, Italy and USA? Why the number of Corona cases in India is increasing? Why so many new cases are coming up everyday? There seems to be something wrong. Let me explain from the beginning. Whatever I am telling you is based on the evidences.

Let me explain from the scratch how a Corona patient is killed in three steps?

Step One

As soon as you get out of the house (in fact, some people even when at home), you put on the face mask thinking that you are protected.

What happens, as reported in a journal[14], in an hour, we touch the mask 23 times on an average.

One tends to adjust the mask, on an average, 23 times in an hour. You go to a shop to buy vegetables putting on the mask. While you are talking to the vendor enquiring the rates, you continuously adjust the mask. Finally, you pick up a fruit let us say, a mango and don't find it up to the mark; you pick up another one; while you are selecting and deselecting the mangoes, your hand again and again goes to the mask, since you are finding it difficult to speak and you are feeling suffocated.

What I am trying to explain is an important thing. Your mouth does not contain only Coronavirus, there are so many types of viruses in your mouth. When you were not using the mask prior to the spread of Corona, on sneezing or coughing, the bacteria and viruses from your mouth used to go into the atmosphere and get killed due to fresh air and sunlight. Now, when you are wearing the mask, you are not letting those bacteria and viruses get killed as there is no fresh air or sunlight; you are, in fact, collecting them in the mask.

Face mask causes stagnation/collection of all kinds of viruses(including Coronavirus) and frequent touching of mask (23 times per hour) causes an increase in the transmission of virus meaning more illness and more deaths.

The first step here is that a healthy human being is sitting at home, away from the sunlight and fresh air; there is no physical activity. A number of people have lost their jobs in this Corona pandemic, so they are depressed; the children are not going to school so even they are depressed; all this is leading to bickering at home. As a result, our immunity gets lowered and whatever immunity we are left with, is lost as a result of the mask. Since you have been continuously adjusting the mask, and touching the mangoes (which you don't buy finally because you don't like them), unintentionally you pass your virus to the mangoes. Another healthy person comes to the shop and buys those mangoes, thereby carrying your virus home (not necessarily Coronavirus, it could be any virus).

For this, I found out all the medical research papers pertaining to whether the mask protects us from virus, Influenza, common cold or not. I succeeded in getting three research papers which were related to the use of masks. One research paper talked about touching the mask 23 times in an hour. The research of other papers[15] was about whether the use of mask alleviates or aggravates the infection. The conclusion of all these research papers was the same. That is, if you use a mask to protect yourself from a particular virus, that virus will increase. So, the first step or conspiracy is to make people sick; to lower their immunity. You are your own immunity. To lower the immunity, make a person sit at home out of fear. The number of times you make a phone call, or read the newspaper or listen to the news, fear will increase leading to the lowering of immunity by about 50%. The remaining immunity is being lowered by the use of masks. Let me ask, "How many times do you wash the mask in a month"? I am pretty sure you don't wash it at all or may be once. The collection of viruses in the mask lowers the immunity and brings it to the same level as the Indian economy currently is (on the verge of crash).

The point that I am trying to emphasize is that the virus, which otherwise would not have come to you, in the prevailing circumstances will come to you and if somebody else's virus comes to you, you would have fought against it in the normal circumstances because your immunity was strong but now with the weak immunity, an otherwise healthy person too would fall sick.

Step Two

Whenever the virus enters your body (because of the use of mask), it is quite obvious that the patient will have cold or cough or fever or some other symptoms. What will the person do in such a case? He will go to the hospital because if he goes to the chemist to buy a medicine for lowering the fever, he will not be given medicine; rather he would be advised to go to the hospital. If you go to the hospital, you will be coerced to undergo Corona test and it is most likely, the report would be positive. Why? This will be discussed later. What follows after being Corona positive, is step 2.

When you reach the hospital, the virus is still in your throat or the upper respiratory tract. Remember till the time the respiratory Influenza virus (Corona) is in the upper respiratory tract, there won't be any complications nor will the person get killed. Respiratory Influenza virus means it can enter the body through the mouth or nose. It remains in the upper respiratory tract for two days. You will catch cold so that the virus comes out or develop fever because at that time, the Coronavirus or for that matter, any virus starts disintegrating, starts getting destroyed and at this time, our immunity throws it out of the body. You will not develop any complications or breathing difficulty because the virus is in the upper respiratory tract and we breathe through the lungs. The virus will go down from the upper respiratory tract after two days if nothing is done to prevent its attack. Gradually, the virus will start going down on the third day onwards when you go to the doctor. The doctor will prescribe antibiotics, anti-pyretic, anti-malarial and anti-HIV medicines.

Coronavirus in upper respiratory tract (mouth, nose, throat) is not at all deadly and cannot cause complication or death.

Giving patients-

1. Antibiotics[16]
2. Antipyretic drugs[17]
3. Anti-viral drugs[18]
4. Anti -malarial drugs[19]

Causes the virus to spread to the lower respiratory tract (Lungs). By 7th day, it may cause breathing difficulties, Pneumonia like symptoms and oxygen deficiency in patients.

Read *Gulf News*[20] of April 9, 2020. This is the reputed newspaper of the Gulf countries wherein my interview was published. The interview says:

"Check the WHO protocol and you will see it's a combination of anti-malarial, antibiotics, anti-pyretics and even in cases a HIV drug. Why do you need antibiotics to treat what is essentially a viral fever? Even the dosage of anti-pyretic is also extremely high and it can often turn out to be a lethal combination."

In many of my interviews, I have indicated that the reason for death is not Coronavirus but the medicines being administered in the name of Coronavirus thus resulting in the movement of the virus to the lungs (lower respiratory tract). All the medicines consumed lower the immunity, as a result the virus gets a chance to percolate down to the lungs. What is helping the virus to move from upper respiratory tract to the lower respiratory tract? Medicines. All this I have been saying since the month of February 2020 because it was happening in Wuhan at that time and it was occurring at other places as well. What was the result? My YouTube channel, Facebook page and Twitter account got deleted.

On June 1, 2020, WHO accepted in *The Guardian*[21] that the overuse of antibiotics for Covid-19 will cause more deaths. What I said 2-3 months back is now being accepted by WHO that the reason for the increased deaths is medicines when so many people have lost their lives, WHO is saying this. You must have noticed that recently the drug for malaria too has been banned because WHO said that it is the reason for increased deaths. The drug for HIV too was banned in the beginning of April for the same reason. WHO is saying all this when so many people have lost their lives? A common man like me also knows that if we intervene with the virus by taking medicines, it will attack the lungs.

Step Three

Once the virus reaches the lungs, fluid is filled up in the alveoli as a result, the patient starts having breathing difficulty. In such a scenario, if you measure the oxygen level with the help of Oximeter, it will be sometimes even less than 80%, which in normal course is 99%. The moment it is < 90%, the doctor would advise you to go on ventilator- step three of murder or death.

See the below given Ventilator. How dangerous the mechanical ventilator looks. It appears that the mechanical ventilator is a life-

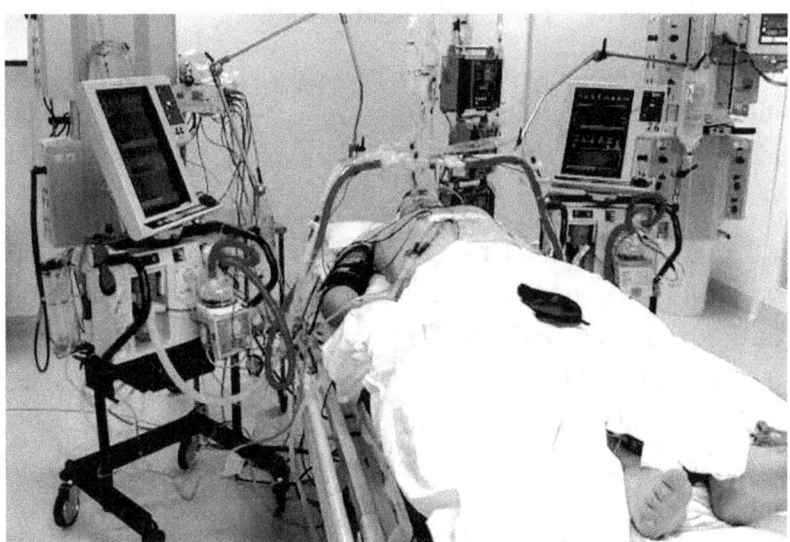

saving equipment. Let me tell you 94% people die on the ventilator[22]. 6% people, who come alive from the ventilator, half of them die within 2-3 months and those 3%, who survive are in a pathetic state i.e. they are dependent on others for their day to day needs. When a person is on ventilator, the ventilator functions as lungs; in such a case, the coordination between the brain and the lungs gets cut off.

What happens after this? When the lungs breathe, the brain does not recognise it and the motor activities such as brushing teeth, eating etc. are forgotten by the body. The person becomes a living corpse. What I am trying to say is that a mechanical ventilator is a trade with death; it is a journey towards death. Based on the evidence, I said 94% deaths occur on the ventilator but my friend, consultant, for N.I.C.E. Dr K B Tumane, Ex-Chief Doctor (Deputy Director Health Services) Nagpur Municipal Corporation, who is a chest specialist for the last 32 years and has been associated with patients suffering from grave diseases of the lungs like Pneumonia, Tuberculosis etc; patients who are in the last stages says that in his long medical career, he has never seen a patient coming alive from the ventilator meaning thereby 100% deaths occur on the ventilator. What he is saying, is practically seen by him.

Thus, the patient dies in three steps. Step one is completed by the mask. Step two is completed when you go the hospital and take medicines and step three is completed by putting the patient on the ventilator.

All over the world, so many deaths are occurring because the protocol is the same (all three steps towards death). Same is the case in India. But India has less number of ventilators so some people are lucky that they do not get admission to the hospital and as a result, they don't get the ventilators and by God's grace, they are saved from death in spite of the doctors and in spite of the treatment. When people ask the reason for the large number of deaths in Brazil or the USA, I got in touch with my network of doctors across the world (from whom I get authentic information) and concluded that whichever country follows the above three steps (Mask, Medicine and Ventilator), the number of deaths is more. In countries like Vietnam (where I have been running my center for the last eight years), Cambodia etc the total number of deaths is zero; in Tanzania, it is 21 deaths out of a total population of six crores; even in Qatar (where I have a large number of patients), the protocol is that people are advised to take rest, keep themselves hydrated and are confined to one room. The entire city or town or the society or the building is not quarantined.

There, whenever a person suffers from Corona, he is isolated (as in any infectious disease) and the rest of the work goes on. The point that I am trying to emphasise is that it is not such a virus, which if attacks, will spread to all.

Since people die in three steps, it is a joint responsibility on our part (both you and me) to save them from death and give them the right knowledge. Right knowledge means if at all the virus enters the body, it should not go beyond the upper respiratory tract. If you succeed in doing this, I assure you that the patient won't die of Corona. Remember we all are born to die, but we won't embrace death by becoming a victim of any disease (here Corona).

What is the solution? This is very important. 60 % of the people in the world are already immune to novel Coronavirus or SARS-CoV-2 the new virus - as if they are already vaccinated against Corona. Despite the absence of the vaccine, they are immune. Research paper of May 14, 2020 in Cell[23]- a reputed and highly regarded journal, says that 60% of the people in the world are immune to Coronavirus. The researchers found that the viruses like the Hong Kong Coronavirus in 2005, the Netherland Coronavirus in 2004 or 229E the US Coronavirus in 1965- all these viruses have given us cold and fever several times; as a result, a type of immunity is developed in our body and this immunity is called Background immunity. 60% of people in the world are having **background immunity.**

Cellular background Immunity: Up to 60% of the population has cellular background immunity to novel Coronavirus as they have been infected with the previous Coronaviruses (cold virus) since childhood.

What about the remaining 40%. They have another type of immunity called **Herd immunity**. In any country or community for that matter, if 60-70% of the population becomes immune, the rest of the population becomes safe. This is due to **Herd immunity.** The day Coronavirus came to light, we (60%) were covered with **Background immunity** and the remaining 40% got covered with **Herd immunity.** Thus, this world is already being protected from novel Coronavirus from the time it entered our country.

Herd Immunity: Since 60% of the population is already having background immunity, rest 40% may get covered partially under herd immunity. Because of it, global case fatality ratio is 0.1% i.e. equal to the seasonal Flu.

How would you recover? Most of our population already has background immunity as well as herd immunity. There is a third type of immunity called **Mucosal immunity**- immunity related to mucus- called a "Chipchipa Padharth" in Ayurveda. Our body is lined with mucus right from the mouth itself. As soon as the virus enters the body, it confronts mucosal immunity at first. If you strengthen your mucosal immunity, you need not worry about respiratory virus. How can you strengthen mucosal immunity? By consuming 0.2 gm Vitamin C[24]. Vitamin C should be taken not in tablet form but by consuming fruit and vegetables- 2 mangoes /

2 sweet limes / 4 tomatoes / a handful of raw peas/different types of fruits (300-400 gm) all give 0.2 gm vitamin C. A vitamin tablet taken goes directly into the stomach whereas the fruits and vegetables consumed orally go to the body through mouth and strengthen the mucosal immunity. Whenever you take a tablet, any tablet for that matter, your mucosal immunity is reduced.

Mucosal Immunity: Everyday consume at least 0.2 gm of vitamin C from fruits (3 mangoes, 2 oranges or 1 guava) raw vegetables (4 tomatoes or a handful of peas) to prevent the attack of respiratory viruses.

Step One

You have three types of immunity; background immunity, herd immunity and mucosal immunity. Strengthen them by consuming 0.2 gm vitamin C, by avoiding the intake of medicines (as they lower the immunity) and reduce (in fact completely avoid) the intake of animal protein (any food derived from animals) such as mutton, chicken, fish, egg, dairy products-milk, curd, butter milk etc. Animal protein reduces mucosal immunity. Despite these three types of immunity, the virus enters the body because the person is on medicines or consuming animal protein, and the person falls sick.

Step Two

As soon as the first sign of Flu like symptoms such as feeling feverish, headache, body ache, cold or cough occur, immediately follow the three days protocol (which I have been prescribing to my patients since 2016).

With the first symptom of Flu (fever, cough, body ache, weakness)

follow the three step Flu diet.[25]

The three step Flu diet works and is based on the evidence from more than 167 research papers from the last 100 years.[26]

Day 1 (Liquid)

Consume citrus fruit juice and coconut water in the quantity specified below:

Your Body Weight (kg)/10 glasses of fresh citrus fruit juice + Body Weight (kg)/10 glasses of coconut water

Let us say the body weight is 60 kg so 60/10 = 6 glasses of citrus fruit juice and 6 glasses of coconut water.

Don't consume packed juice instead have fresh juice and take it without sieving. Take juice and coconut water alternately every hour, sip by sip, spending at least 15 minutes on each glass. This will keep the temperature under control. Vitamin C in citrus fruit juice supports the immunity and helps in getting rid of the virus. Coconut water helps in hydration. It is the best mineral water in the world made by God.

Day 2 (Fluid)

Consume citrus fruit juice and coconut water

Body Weight (kg) /20 glasses of citrus fruit juice + Body Weight (kg) /20 glasses of coconut water

+

Your Body Weight (kg) × 5 gm of cucumber and tomatoes.

Let us say the body weight is 60 kg so 60/20= 3 glasses of citrus fruit juice and 3 glasses of coconut water

And 60 × 5 =300 gm of cucumber and tomatoes

You will be surprised to see that by the end of Day 2, you start feeling better and your temperature is under control. You would have regained some strength.

Day 3 (Solid)

For breakfast, consume

Body Weight (kg)/30 glasses of citrus fruit juice + Body Weight (kg)/30 glasses of coconut water

If your body weight is 60 kg so 60/30= 2 glasses of citrus fruit juice and 2 glasses of coconut water.

For lunch, consume

Your Body Weight (kg) × 5 gm of cucumber and tomatoes

If your body weight is 60 kg, so 60 × 5 =300 gm of cucumber and tomatoes

By evening, you will be surprised to find yourself fit. You can have normal home cooked food with less oil, less salt leaving animal protein for dinner.

If you follow this simple diet, you would be back to work on the fourth day.

Step Three

Usually, people try to manage the Flu with medicines and sometimes, there are chances for the virus to move down from the upper respiratory tract to the lower respiratory tract. As a result, breathing difficulty occurs and if checked with Oximeter, the oxygen level comes out to be ≤ 90%. In such a situation, the doctor advises a ventilator because the lungs are full of water. What you have to do in such a situation is avoid going to the hospital because you would be put on mechanical ventilator. You have to make your own ventilator at home. This is called Prone ventilation[27]. In the later chapter, I will tell you about Prone Ventilation.

The N.I .C.E INITIATIVE

With the first sign of Flu, contact us at www.biswaroop.com/nice or call us at 8587059169 for free support, guidance and treatment. It is an absolutely free service.

Thereafter, immediately our network of people will contact the patient and guide him. We will be with the person till he comes out of the web of Corona/Flu/Influenza.

References :

To access the references and videos related to this chapter, go to the link www.biswaroop.com/nicebook

---

CHAPTER-3

The Science of Prana-Yamraaj

(Based on the lecture delivered on June 21, 2020-International Yoga Day)

What is SARS-CoV-2?

SARS-CoV-2 is an RNA respiratory Influenza virus. RNA respiratory influenza virus means that it can enter the human body through mouth and nose only. It is an RNA Influenza virus meaning that there can be no medicine or vaccine for the same. The reason for this is that it mutates very easily and quickly. Recently on May 5, 2020, University College of London conducted a study[28] of this virus on 7500 people and came to realize that the virus had already mutated 198 times by then.

Thus it can very safely be said that ever since the virus started spreading from Wuhan, it must have already mutated thousands of times (even though, there is no evidence to prove that the virus did not exist before Wuhan, as explained in the first chapter). Mutation means that it keeps changing its form like an impersonator and that it cannot be found in the same state next time when we reach out for it. Hence, for such viruses which mutate so fast, there can be no medicine or vaccine.

Let's take an example:

If a wild boar comes running towards you and you pick up a weapon to kill it but, as soon as you pick up the weapon, the boar turns into a mosquito. Now, that weapon cannot be used to kill the mosquito. As soon as the weapon is changed, the mosquito turns into an elephant. A mutant virus is of similar type. It keeps changing its form. Hence, this RNA Influenza virus is also of mutant type. When 7500 people were tested, it was found that the virus had already mutated 198 times. If a larger sample is collected, then, we would find that the virus has mutated thousands and lakhs of times. Thus it is clear that if some virus is prone to excessive mutation, no medicine or vaccine can be created for it. By the time the medicine is created, it would be into some other form.

Secondly, nobody can die due to Coronavirus infection. The reason for this is very simple. This virus enters the body through the mouth and the nose. Till the time it is in the upper respiratory tract, there can be no complications or harm. After 4-5 days, it reaches the lower respiratory tract, where it can cause Pneumonia, ARDS (Acute Respiratory Distress Syndrome) or even cardiac injury. Plenty of people have succumbed to Covid-19 infection which occurs only when the virus moves to the lower respiratory tract.

Why does the virus come down to lower respiratory tract? I have explained it earlier also that in case you suffer from Covid-19 infection, Flu or Influenza and at such a time, if you take medicine like any antibiotic, antipyretic, anti -malaria, anti- HIV or any other medicine for that matter, it directly or indirectly compromises with your immunity and the virus gets an opportunity to travel from the upper respiratory tract to the lower respiratory tract. This can lead to Pneumonia or any other breathing problem. At such a time, conventionally, the first thing is administering of oxygen and next comes the mechanical ventilator. People feel that if they are put on the ventilator, they will survive but let me tell you that the ventilator has a failure ratio of up to 94%. This mechanical machine, which is called the ventilator, is actually a bane for humanity because the pipe which goes through the throat down to the lungs and tries to pump oxygen, at that moment, the connection between the brain and the lungs is snapped. The patient, who is put on the ventilator, finally has difficulty in coordinating the brain with the actions of the body and therefore, we see him in the conditions which are so disturbing.

Let me remind you that today is International Yoga Day and yoga is something which we Indians have given to the world and this asana that is Pranayam- the breathing exercise-shows the connection between the lungs and the brain. It is the lungs which control the breathing and when this connection between the brain and the lungs is snapped, then the mind-body coordination is ruined. At that moment, the patient is alive but like a dead body. The breathing is on but the brain does not know who he is. This is what is done by the mechanical ventilator.

Hence, people who survive on ventilator, are actually living corpses. So, the ventilator is not a boon for humanity. You would very well understand this if you have met a person or a patient who was ever put on a ventilator.

Today, if somebody has tested positive for Coronavirus and he goes to the hospital the charges for the bed in the hospital range from Rs 3-4 or even Rs 5 lakhs. It might even range to Rs 25 lakhs which might (for some) mean the entire earning of their lives. Imagine your entire earnings for just one bed in the hospital. Let me now ask a valid question-What do you get out of that bed in the hospital? If there is no medicine for Coronavirus, no vaccine then, what is the point in getting admitted to the hospitals and spending 7 to 10 lakhs? One must ask oneself, "What is it that the doctor is going to treat me with?", as till date, there isn't any medicine or vaccine or machine which can help the Covid-19 patients. The hospitals have nothing which can increase the chances of survival even by a fraction. In addition, they do have certain things which might enhance the chances of death.

Let me now assure you that it is actually very simple to be cured of this virus especially with the three day Flu diet for SARS-CoV-2 is a harmless Flu virus and is rarely fatal. People generally question why so many deaths are reported in India? The answer is quite straight forward. Rather than Corona being the culprit, the real contributor to the death toll is the treatment protocol by the WHO (as explained earlier) and the change in guidelines of "reporting death" by ICMR.

ICMR recently issued guidelines that if anybody died on the Indian soil and was suffering from breathing difficulty or had cardiac injury then that would be considered death due to Coronavirus even if he or she tested negative for Corona. Now, can you tell me about anyone who would not be having breathing difficulty or cardiac injury at the time of death? Whenever a person dies, two things are always there: one is breathing difficulty and another one is cardiac problem i.e. the heart stops and the breathing stops. Both these conditions were cited by ICMR to be considered as Corona deaths. Also, in accordance to the changed guidelines, if a patient died of accident and also tested Corona positive, it is to be considered as death due to Coronavirus. Thus the deaths in India include all these patients as well. Honestly speaking, no one knows correctly how many patients really died of Coronavirus. My personal experience with Coronavirus patients is that if you give such a person comfort and keep the patient hydrated, then Coronavirus would vanish in 3 to 5 days. It is just like any other Flu.

It is not difficult to predict the behaviour of the newly discovered SARS-CoV-2 (however, it may be infecting humans since eternity), as four other Coronaviruses (229E, NL63, OC43, HKU1) were already known to human beings for several years and also statistically about 10% of the Flu, which we suffered in our lifetime, is the result of the invasion of one of the above kind of Coronaviruses and each time we get cured, without much effort and attention, in just a span of three to seven days.

Let us say somebody wants to eat a mango. The mango has the same features be it any part of the world. They might vary in size, shape and taste but the basic things would be the same. Similarly, this Covid-19 is essentially the same as the other four viruses. The fatality rate and the means of transmission would basically remain the same. Thus, we can conclude that even this virus would be similar in behaviour to the other four, so there is nothing to fear about.

Let us look at the example of Vietnam where I have been practising for the last seven years. Coronavirus had reached Vietnam much before it reached India and let me tell you that the number of deaths in Vietnam due to Coronavirus is zero. No one died in Vietnam due to Coronavirus. I asked my Vietnamese colleagues about the zero Corona deaths in Vietnam. The answer that they gave was, "Our country does not experiment with drugs on human beings. We just advise the patients to take complete rest and they soon recover."

Vietnam has a population of about 15-16 crore and still it has no deaths whereas in India, the entire economy is shattered and the people are living under the scare of Corona. On the occasion of International Yoga Day, it is quite unfortunate (since it is solar eclipse also) the newspaper headlines have flashed the launch of 'Fabi Flu'. This drug is an experimental drug and there is no explanation of what harm it would do once it reaches the body. None of the countries including US, UK and Japan (where it was developed in 2014) have approved of it but India has approved of it as an experimental drug. The launch of this drug may, God forbid, announce a total eclipse for India.

Whenever a new medicine is launched in the market, there is some reference or clinical trial to decide that this medicine will be beneficial for a particular ailment. When I tried to find the clinical trial reference of Fabi Flu (Favipiravir), I got just one trial and that too, had come from China a few months back. On the one hand, we are boycotting Chinese goods and people are being motivated not to use Chinese products and on the other hand, the trial from China is considered as a reference for launching this medicine. I studied this trial wherein 80 patients were involved; 35 patients were given Favipiravir medicine, which is launched by the name-Fabi Flu. 45 people were given another medicine named Lopinavir and Ritonavir. These two are the failed drugs of HIV which were given to the patients in the name of Corona. These drugs were banned when the number of deaths started increasing. So the banned drugs are being compared to this new medicine Fabi Flu. This is similar to a cunning boy who fails in the class. He gets only 20 marks but wants to inform his parents that he has got very good marks so he brings home another child who got just 10 marks. He wants to tell his parents that my marks may be bad but there is someone whose marks are worse. In the same fashion, this trial proves that this medicine is better than Lopinavir and Ritonavir. It does not show that this medicine can cure a Corona patient. A careful study of this trial shows that it is neither a randomized control trial nor a double blinded trial. People who conducted the trial chose and decided to keep the patients in this category of medicine (Fabi Flu) or that (Lopinavir and Ritonavir). The 35 patients of Fabi Flu category were thin, young, less sick and their temperature was lower in comparison to the patients of the other group. Some of them were even asymptomatic. Thus, the seriously ill Covid-19 patients were excluded, so it cannot be considered a real trial.

In order to know the truth of this medicine, have a look at this manual[29] which I have taken from the Ministry of Health, Labour and Welfare, Japan dated March 4, 2014, when Fabi Flu was made. Read this manual and you would get to know the entire truth. On Page 56 of this manual, it is written that this medicine was tried on 12 puppies, out of which nine puppies died in a few days. Then, the medicine was tried on three monkeys; one monkey died in a few days. After this, the medicine was tried on some rats. As a result, the male rats got testes toxicity meaning they became infertile or impotent. The female rats lost their ability to produce young ones. Thus, either still born children were being produced or they were being born with genetic defects. Such medicines are assigned a special category referred to as teratogenic drugs. How harmful are teratogenic drugs, I will explain by referring to an article in the *New York Times*[30] of May 6, 2020. The article says that this medicine (Fabi Flu) can be compared to another teratogenic drug called Thalidomide launched in 1950 in some European nations. The side effects of this drug were that 1,23,000 children were still born. Those who were born alive suffered from deformities of various kinds. (See picture)

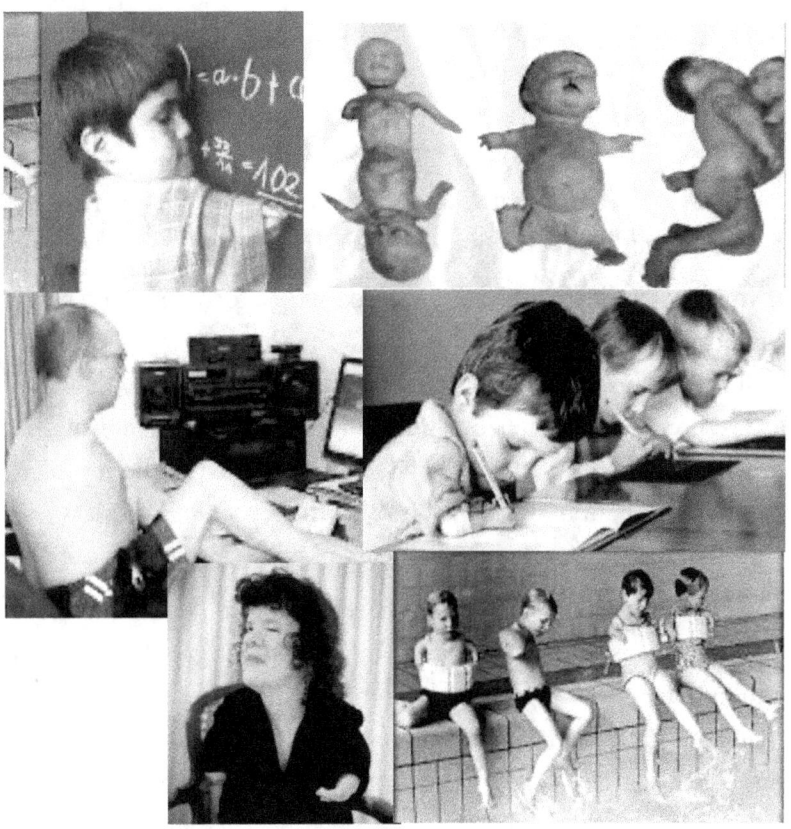

There are around 24000 such children who are still living with those disabilities. Thus this medicine was soon banned. Similar condition may arise with this drug i.e. 'Fabi Flu'. The side effects would be known after some years. The newspapers and the drug companies might hide the side effects but they will be out very soon when the children are born.

Fabi Flu in India

Let us discuss Fabi Flu in the Indian context. On June 20, 2020, when this medicine was launched in India, the newspapers and TV revealed its price as INR 103. People think by consuming medicine worth INR 103, they will recover from Corona. The truth is that the full strip of medicine (containing 34 tablets) is to be consumed on the very first day. In 14 days, 7-8 such strips of medicines are to be consumed, meaning thereby one has to consume tablets worth INR 25000 in 14 days to recover. The recovery will be only for those people who are already fine (asymptomatic). What will be its effect on the seriously ill patients is not known.

If you buy this medicine, you need to fill up a form, inserted inside the box. You need to sign this form. The form says that you have well understood the side effects of this medicine and you yourself are responsible for the side effects; no one else. After consuming the medicine, how it affects, that data will be taken by the company, compiled and put in the next edition of the report just as this report explains the effect of this medicine on puppies, monkeys and rats.

The next report of this medicine is very likely to describe its effect on the Indians. This is known as human guinea pig. Human trial and human guinea pig are two different things. Human trial means that a person has given consent to become a part of the trial (for his vested interests- may be for financial gains). Such people get

INR10-15 lakh. The person becomes willing to take a chance. This is known as volunteer for human trial. The other is guinea pig which means that you buy these medicines for INR 25000 and become a part of the trial. You will become like the puppies or monkeys or rats. This is called human guinea pig.

The trial pertaining to how this medicine will work on Corona patients, never took place. Only comparison was made that this medicine better than the other two medicines as it was tried on almost asymptomatic patients.

I suggest, download the manual (consisting of 172 pages) of this medicine and read it thoroughly. Then go to any doctor or health specialist and ask him if any near and dear one in his family (may be his kid/ wife/ parents) or even he himself gets Covid-19, will he prescribe this medicine?

As stated earlier, Coronavirus is an RNA respiratory Influenza virus and it mutates fast so there can be no drug for the same. This drug, which is available in the market, brings about genetic changes. It genetically changes or mutates the RNA of the body. Putting it simply, you become an entirely different person although the body remains the same; in other words, it shakes the foundations of the human body so in the near future, there are chances that the person might suffer from autoimmune diseases or Cancer or tumour. This might not happen to you but to the forthcoming generations. What all can it possibly do is shown to you through the photographs on the previous page. So be careful while you take this drug. It is not that the regulating authorities do not know about this drug; none of the countries have launched it commercially except India. The Indian economy has already been paralyzed and now schemes are on to paralyze the citizens of India.

On the occasion of the International Yoga Day, let's talk of yoga. Pranayam is an important exercise in which oxygen reaches those parts of body (where it normally doesn't) through the medium of short breaths or longer deep ones. This leads to curing of or prevention of the diseases like Cancer, Diabetes and other such ailments. Plenty of people in and around the world follow yogic exercises specially Pranayam. I can safely say that Pranayam or breathing exercise alone is one holistic cure. If we do the reverse of it, that is, if we, instead of allowing oxygen to reach the cells of the body, make carbon dioxide reach them, then, what would happen and if this process continues for long hours and on daily basis, then of course, one would say that the reverse would be true. If this is followed then, all those diseases like Cancer, Diabetes, Hypertension, Blood Pressure, cardiac diseases etc would also increase. These are the long term effects. What about the short-term problems? It will cause headaches, feeling of fever, loss of immunity etc.

To convey a message, I have found a new method that is- this is a placard which reads **'Pranayam'** and I wear a mask which writes **'Raj'** together it makes **"Prana-yamraj'**.

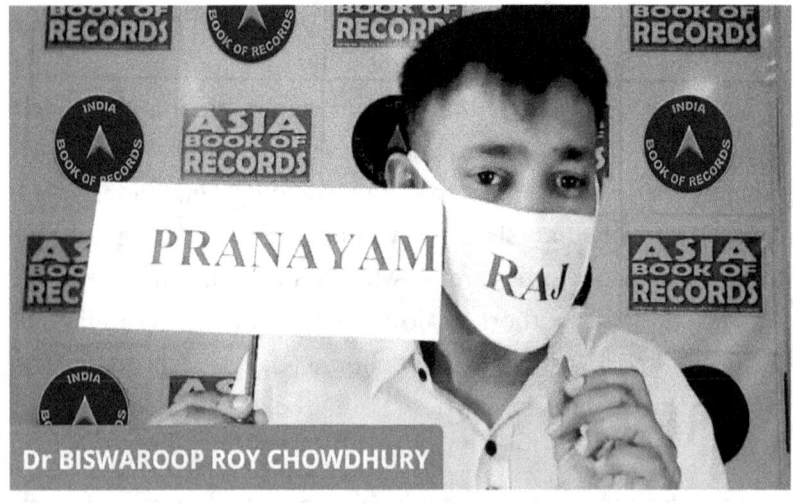

There is a need to understand this clearly. When we wear a mask and we keep breathing, we actually are taking in the carbon dioxide that we ourselves are releasing and it is being done continuously. Those who are healthy would experience the side effects in about an hour or two and those who suffer from co-morbidity will experience this quickly say in about half an hour. Actually, we are opening a channel to reach the Yamraj- God of death.

Look at the report[30] of CDC dated June 10, 2020 (CDC is Centre of Disease Control).They have accepted in this report that if we wear a face mask for more than one hour, it will have physiological effects on the wearer since we take in the carbon dioxide which we ourselves release. It may lead to problems like headache, increased pressure inside the skull, changes in the nervous system, increased breathing frequency, cardiovascular effects, reduced tolerance to lighter workloads etc. I have been emphasising this for the past so many months, and now CDC has accepted it but it is quite unfortunate that our government is not paying any heed to it.

It is noticed from the calls of the patients received in the past few days, that they have complaints of headache, breathing problems and they suspect that they have acquired Coronavirus. I basically tell them to remove their masks and breathe comfortably for 4-5 hours and believe me, they start feeling better. It is important to understand- from where has this 'mask theory' come in. It has basically reached us from the surgeons. While operating, they generally use the masks. We must get into the real scenario whether wearing of mask really helps the surgeon? This culture of wearing masks is 130 years old. There is basically a tradition to wear the mask while performing surgeries and it is strictly followed by the surgeons but whether it is helpful or not is doubtful.

A meta-analysis[31] was done by Cochrane Collaboration. They analysed all the researches made on the simple question whether wearing the mask during surgery is beneficial or performing surgery without the mask is also equally good. This organisation is an unbiased organisation and it never takes donations from any pharmaceutical companies but keeps bringing out the truth. The Cochrane Collaboration continuously researched to find out whether it is beneficial for the surgeons to perform surgeries wearing the mask or is it not beneficial. They gathered all the randomised control trials and came to the conclusion that by wearing the mask, the chances of infection will not be lessened rather they will be increased. Infection does not come down by wearing the mask even during surgeries.

How is the chance of infection increased by wearing the masks?

When we wear a mask and breathe into it then the area (which is covering the nose and the mouth) has the same temperature as our body. Along with this, as we are speaking and breathing at the same moment, this area becomes a little moist or humid. Two things that need to be focussed on here are that this area gets a little warm as well as humid. Humidity and warmth are very conducive atmosphere for germs, bacteria and other infections to flourish. If you wear a mask for half an hour to one hour continuously then, the atmosphere created at this juncture becomes very conducive for the prosperity and growth of infections and germs. The report[32] of the journal-*J. Orthop Translate* of the year 2018 writes about-'Surgical masks as a source of bacterial contamination during operative procedures.'

Thus, by wearing the mask the chances of infection do not decrease rather they increase. The wearing of masks leads to another disease in the human body called 'Hypercapnia'[33] which is the condition where our body has more of carbon dioxide than required. Just as Pranayam means filling the body with oxygen, the reverse of it is

Hypercapnia - that is filling the body with carbon dioxide.

"Hypercapnia alters expression of immune response, nucleosome assembly and lipid metabolism genes in differentiated human bronchial epithelial cells."

-Scientific Reports 2018

The question arises where did this idea of wearing a mask evolve from? It evolved 130 years ago but who is the person who got this idea of making a mask? It came to light that there was a surgeon named Dr Joseph Lister. He was a surgeon in 1880s and was of the opinion that if we wear a mask, we would be safe from infections. Almost all of us are aware of Listerine mouthwash. This product is based on the name of Dr Joseph Lister. Many of us use it as a mouthwash to kill the bad bacteria or viruses in the mouth. It has high alcohol content so the reality is that it does not just kills the harmful bacteria but also the beneficial bacteria which boost our mucosal immunity.

"The role of alcohol in oral carcinogenesis with particular reference to alcohol containing mouthwashes"

-Australian Dental Journal, 2008

Australian Dental Journal of 2008 published a report[34] saying it causes Cancer. Both these ideas i.e. one of wearing the mask and the other of using mouthwashes (alcohol- based mouthwashes) evolved from the same person-Dr Joseph Lister.

We are surrounded by bacteria and viruses and millions of them live inside our body. We live in harmony with them. To throw out the bad bacteria or viruses or any other infection from the body is the duty of our immune system. This immunity exists everywhere- in the mouth, skin and everywhere else. We kill the immunity in our mouth by the use of alcohol- based mouthwashes and we kill the immunity of our hands by using alcohol -based sanitizers. The truth is that both mouthwashes and hand washes are the same because the ingredients of both are almost the same and both of them are cancerous. They are the substances which actually depress the immunity and while we require immunity to fight for our safety, these are the products which lower it. Remember that those people who are trying to promote sanitizers and mouthwashes or even over cleanliness are actually promoting Cancer.

What needs to be done? The solution

'N.I.C.E'- is a network of Influenza Care Experts in which we have about 200 experts from around the country. We often encounter patients with complaints of feverishness, headache or weakness; they might be suffering from Flu or Coronavirus or even Influenza but the basic reason can also be that they have worn the mask for a longer time. Let's perform an experiment. Take an Oximeter and check your oxygen level and your pulse rate. After checking these two things, wear your mask for about an hour and then once again, check your oxygen level and pulse rate. You will find that your pulse rate has increased by 5 or 7 units. It means that wearing the mask directly affects your heart and therefore, the pulse rate increases. What is the effect of mask on oxygen level? If a person wears the mask for half an hour, the oxygen level reduces by 1%. This is confirmed through the research paper[35] published in *Neurocirugia* in 2008. You can always perform the experiment yourself and find out the result.

In our vicinity, we have so many health workers, policemen, shopkeepers etc and other people who, because of their duty, have to continuously wear masks for long hours. If they do not wear the masks, they will be fined for non- compliance. When such people contact us and tell us that they have symptoms like headache, fever, weakness and breathing problems, the same symptoms as that of Covid-19, We ask them to remove the masks, we know that wearing of mask also leads to the same problems. Diagnosis of such patients show- low oxygen saturation level, increase in pulse rate and temperature. The low saturation level of oxygen in such patients can lead to Pneumonia, due to increased pulse rate; they can suffer cardiac injury and due to high temperature, they can feel feverish and weak. Although the temperature increases only by half a degree but that half degree will remain in the increased position for longer durations, which can be highly risky.

SYMPTOM	COVID-19	MASK
Headache	√	√
Breathing difficulty	√	√
Weakness	√	√
DIAGNOSIS		
Oxygen	↓	↓
Pulse	↑	↑
Temperature	↑	↑

Here I would like to reiterate the fact that wearing the mask and breathing into it leads to about half a degree increase in the body temperature. Here the relation is with the thermoregulation of the body. 'Face mask impact on human thermoregulation', this article is recently published in *The Annals of Occupational Hygiene 2020*. On reading the article[36], you will understand that the brain, which regulates the entire body temperature, gets disturbed because of wearing the mask; as a result, the temperature of the body increases by up to half a degree. Although, half a degree is a very mild increase but it remains like this for a longer duration of time. This long-standing increase can be quite dangerous for the human body. If you have Flu like symptoms, they may not be the symptoms of Coronavirus or Influenza; in fact, they are due to the lack of oxygen in your body.

In case you have certain patients around you who have Covid-19 like symptoms, you can tell them that these symptoms can be because of wearing the mask or you may even suggest them the three step Flu diet which has been explained earlier in the book. If they are still not confident, you can connect them to us through our helpline number. Those people who are MBBS doctors or BHMS or BMS or even Health Care workers, I invite you to support us and help us by joining N.I.C.E.

You can join us on our website www.biswaroop.com/expert. I will provide you special training as to how to handle Influenza/ Covid-19 patients. With your background knowledge, you can be a part of this network and we can together help people recover from Covid-19 /Flu.

References :

To access the references and videos related to this chapter, go to the link : www.biswaroop.com/nicebook

CHAPTER-4

Emergency Management
of ILI/Covid-19

(Based on "The Training for N.I.C.E. Practitioners" held on June 29, 2020)

Emergency Management of ILI/ Covid-19
1) Breathing Management
2) Cough Management
3) Fever Management
4) Vomiting
5) Nausea
6) Extreme Weakness
7) Loose Motion

The most important thing while managing the Flu/Influenza/ILI/ Covid-19 is managing the following symptoms like breathing, cough, fever, vomiting, nausea and extreme weakness. In such a situation, the patients might panic; we need to remind them that they need to keep some patience; that is why they are called patients. We need to ask them only two things: the temperature and the SpO2 i.e. the oxygen level using Oximeter. As long as the temperature is ≤ 102°F, it is okay. If the oxygen level is ≥ 88%, then it is comfortable.

Let's start with breathing management. Breathing management means the person is finding difficulty in breathing. For such a person, we think of oxygen in the hospital set up. If the breathing difficulty persists, then we think of mechanical ventilator. Oxygen cylinder or oxygen therapy is the worst fraud in the medical industry. Why? Because your body is not designed to take in pure oxygen. Your body is designed to inhale air which has only 21% oxygen and the rest are nitrogen and other gases. This is an important thing, which you should keep in mind.

For example, you have a petrol or a diesel car. Instead of petrol or diesel, you put more purified and more expensive fuel that is, the jet fuel, do you think the car will run? The answer is no. Your car is designed for petrol/diesel. Even if you put superior kind of fuel, it is not going to work. The engine will be damaged. Similarly, your body is not designed to inhale oxygen for a long time or even for a minute. It is going to damage your body. The very thought that oxygen therapy can help a person to reduce the mortality/morbidity, is untrue. Ever since the oxygen therapy was introduced in this world, there has not been even a single evidence, which shows that oxygen therapy can increase the life expectancy or it can help save a person's life. No doubt, on providing oxygen therapy, a person may get initial comfort but if you think it is going to increase your life span, it is going to help reduce the morbidity; it is going to help cure the disease, there is no evidence.

I am going to show you the evidence and then you would believe- that is Cochrane Systematic Review-one evidence that I trust the most and I often talk about. Cochrane is an organisation which does not take any donation from any pharmaceutical company. They did a meta analysis[37]- the highest of all kinds of analyses. According to Cochrane, two groups of people were taken-one was given higher concentration of oxygen and the other was given lower concentration of oxygen. Those who were given higher concentration suffered more harm; those who received lower concentration suffered less harm. So lower concentration of oxygen is better.

Higher v/s Lower Oxygen

Higher versus lower fraction of inspired oxygen or targets of arterial oxygenation for adults admitted to the intensive care unit

Cochrane Systematic Review – 27 November 2019

If you ask a question oxygen, or no oxygen – which is better? No oxygen is better than some oxygen. Here is the reference[38]. In the hospital set up, there is an oxygen cylinder which can provide some initial comfort but the same thing you can achieve at home with a hand held fan. The trick is very simple. A hand held fan is available in almost every home. You just have to hold it in front of the nose of the patient. Switch on the fan and the fan will throw air into the nose of the patient. If the patient can hold the fan in front of his nose for 5 minutes (see pic), he will get the same kind of comfort which he might have received with oxygen therapy in the hospital. This will be without the side effects of oxygen which causes oxygen toxicity in the body. A hand held fan is much better than oxygen therapy.

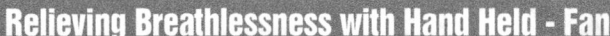

Relieving Breathlessness with Hand Held - Fan

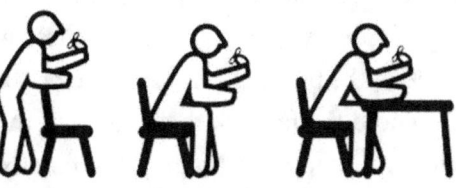

European Respiratory Journal 2017 50: 1701383;
DOI: 10.1183/13993003.01383-2017

Lancet is one among the top five journals. If an article is published in *Lancet,* it is considered as a highly regarded research paper. It is a double-blind randomized controlled trial and here the researchers compared two groups of people who were suffering from breathlessness of similar kind of intensity. One group was given oxygen and the second one was given a fan like this and asked to hold it six inches away from their nose. They were asked to breathe through the air of the fan. Both the groups of people got the same kind of comfort after 5 minutes of these therapies. Thus it is clearly established that this fan can do the same job as an oxygen cylinder. This fan is much cheaper (costing nearly Rs 200) than the oxygen cylinder which is not available at home and for which, we are dependent on the hospital.

Oxygen v/s Room Air in Breathlessness

Effect of palliative oxygen versus medical (room) air in relieving breathlessness in patients with refractory dyspnoea: a double-blind randomized controlled trial

Cochrane Systematic Review – 27 November 2019

The hospital authorities would never say that this fan is better than the oxygen cylinder for fear of their business being severely affected. So for 95% of the patients, who complain of breathlessness, if you ask them to hold the fan like this and sit in this posture (by leaning a little forward and then holding the fan six inches away from their nose), they will get the same comfort as they would have got from the oxygen cylinder. There is no upper limit and they can hold the fan till they get comfort. This is a very important therapy; it is widely written in the medical journals but never shared with the general public. Once it is shared with the general public, they would know that they don't require oxygen cylinder at all. By doing this, you would succeed in solving 95% of your patient's problems.

There are remaining 5% people, who would not get relief despite holding the fan even for half an hour or more. They are the patients who may have the real problem. At this point of time, you could check their SpO2 i.e. oxygen saturation level with the help of Oximeter. If the reading is ≤ 88%, that means it is a real problem-uncontrolled breathlessness -it means it is real emergency and in hospital set up, they are asked to go for mechanical ventilator. What is mechanical ventilator and what is its alternate? The alternative will not provide the same results as mechanical ventilator but far better results than the mechanical ventilator.

Breathing (Emergency Management)	
Hospital	**Home**
Oxygen Cylinder	**Hand Held Fan**
⬇	⬇
Mechanical Ventilators	**Prone Ventilators**

Put the patient on prone ventilation for half an hour and again check the SpO2 and you will find it ≥ 90% and the patient will also start feeling better.

Before focusing on prone ventilation, let me tell you why to avoid mechanical ventilator.

The mechanical ventilator- something very huge, looks very scientific, something very promising, something very glamorous in a way that it is very expensive and not everyone can afford and this is a status symbol of the hospital- a person feels that it is something as modern as this- the hospital has more capacity of saving a person- but this is all glamour.

A ventilator simply means a pipe goes from your nose and mouth to the lungs and stomach. Here the feeding is done through the pipe in the nose and air goes to the lungs through the mouth. This means the person is totally dependent on the pipes as shown in the figure.

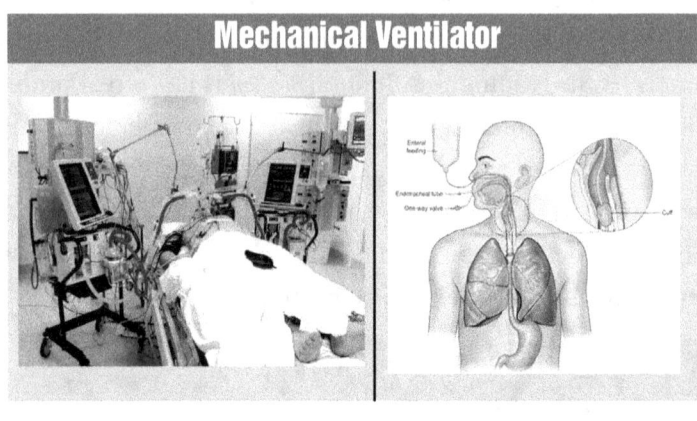

Put on ventilator, 9 in 10 Covid-19 patients die

April 23, 2020   Live Science

When too may pipes go into the body, they give rise to many ailments. It is seen that nine out of ten Covid-19 patients, who are put on the ventilator never come back from the ventilator. They die. One patient survives not because of the ventilator but he survives in spite of being put on the ventilator. So, the patient may be lucky or extremely unlucky. Unlucky because staying on the ventilator is very painful; secondly, those who come out are in a pathetic state and die within next 2-3 months and still those who survive are paralyzed till death relieves them. Why is it so?

Side Effects of Mechanical Ventilator

Mechanical Ventilator

1. VALI (Ventilator Associated Lung Injury)
2. Oxygen Toxicity
3. Neuro Damage
4. VAP (Ventilator Associated Pneumonia)

When the patients are on the ventilator, they get VALI (Ventilator Associated Lung Injury) i.e. through the ventilator, the oxygen is forced on the lungs at a particular speed. Since our body is not designed to take the stream of oxygen at any speed, it immediately damages the lungs, which were already compromised at the first place. Secondly, putting on the ventilator causes oxygen toxicity. As stated earlier, our body is not designed to take in pure oxygen but through ventilator the oxygen is given in pure form. The speed and the purity of oxygen together cause neuro damage. The brain and the lungs, which are in tune with each other and work in harmony with each other, lose the connection with each other after the person is put on the ventilator. As a result, the person loses his memory and cannot perform simple skills like brushing teeth, going to the toilet, eating food, holding the glass etc. He becomes like a small child and needs to relearn all these skills. In extreme cases, the person suffers from VAP (Ventilator Associated Pneumonia). Try to understand this. When a number of pipes go into your body, the bacteria and virus travel through the pipe and occupy a place in the inner part of the lungs. This is called Ventilator Associated Pneumonia and when the person dies, he dies of Pneumonia and not of Influenza or Covid-19 but unfortunately, it is categorised as Corona death. Thus these are the ailments a patient is destined to get when put on a mechanical ventilator.

Role of Bacteria as a cause of death in Pandemic Influenza

J Infect Dis. 2018 October 1; 198(7): 962-970. doi: 10.1086/591708

The Solution: Prone Ventilation

Whenever a person is hospitalised and is on medication or ventilator and dies, the death is not due to Pneumonia caused by virus but Pneumonia caused due to bacteria. The virus makes way for the bacteria. What I am trying to emphasise is that if the virus stays in the body for longer periods, it makes way for the bacteria especially through the ventilator. The bacteria travel through the pipes and go to the lungs, which have numerous small balloon like sacs called alveoli. These sacs are filled with oxygen and exchange of gases takes place here. Now the bacteria occupy these sacs and fill them with liquid thus resulting in breathlessness.

To solve this problem, look at fig -1.

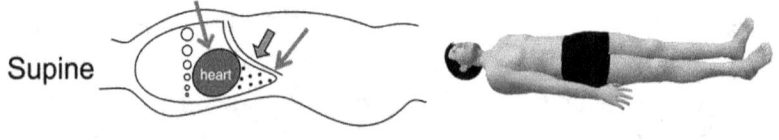

Supine

Figure-1

This is the way we normally lie down (with face up). The small dots represent the sacs/alveoli, which are about 50 crore in number. In this position, the gravitational pressure of heart and the gravitational pressure of abdomen lie on the corner of the lungs and as a result, the balloons squeeze in size thereby about 20% capacity of the lungs is reduced. A healthy human being has no effect with the 20% reduction in the lungs capacity but when one is sick (since 20% is compromised), it affects him badly. If we can take away the gravitational pressure of the heart and the abdomen, then we can utilize that 20%. For this, we need to change the posture, it is called prone positioning or **prone ventilation**. As you can see in fig -2,

the small balloons become bigger in size and this increases the capacity of the lungs by about 20% and that is the distance between life and death. The person, who was earlier on the verge of death, now survives.

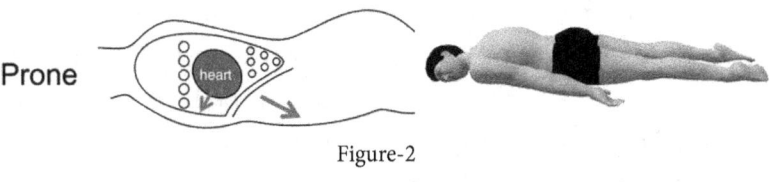

Figure-2

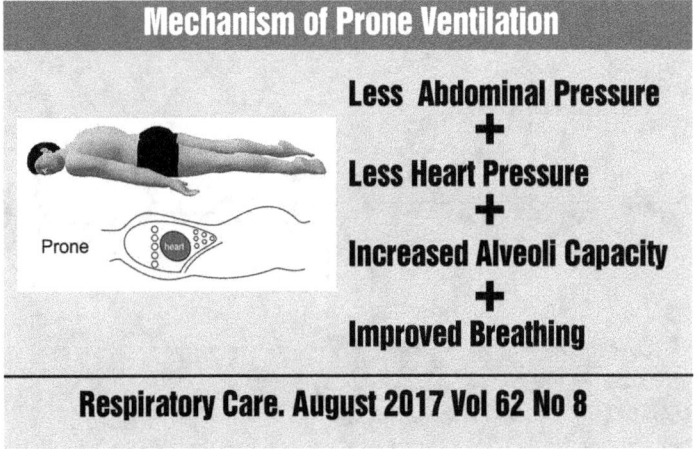

Prone ventilation has been in practice since 1970s. In the last one decade or so, when the mechanical ventilator became popular, prone ventilation and other such things were sidelined to promote the sale of mechanical ventilator and for material gains. Prone ventilation has no side effects as compared to the mechanical ventilator, which has four dangerous side effects resulting in nine deaths out of ten. On May 15, 2020, in the *Journal of American Medical Association*, researchers examined 500 or more Covid-19 patients, who were put on Prone ventilation, no one died. All of them survived. Thus, on the one hand is mechanical ventilator, which is very expensive and painful and causes most of the deaths and on the other hand, is Prone ventilation which can be done at home and has no side effects and the cure rate is 100% especially for Covid-19 patients.

To conclude, when you put a person on Prone ventilation, the abdominal as well as the heart pressure are less, there is increased alveoli capacity and thus improved breathing. All this is expected in about half an hour. But here the recommendation is that the patient should be in Prone ventilation posture for at least 12 hours in a day because the moment he gets up, the breathing problem would start. He may take a break of 10-15 minutes every hour. During the break, he can move his body and be in any posture.

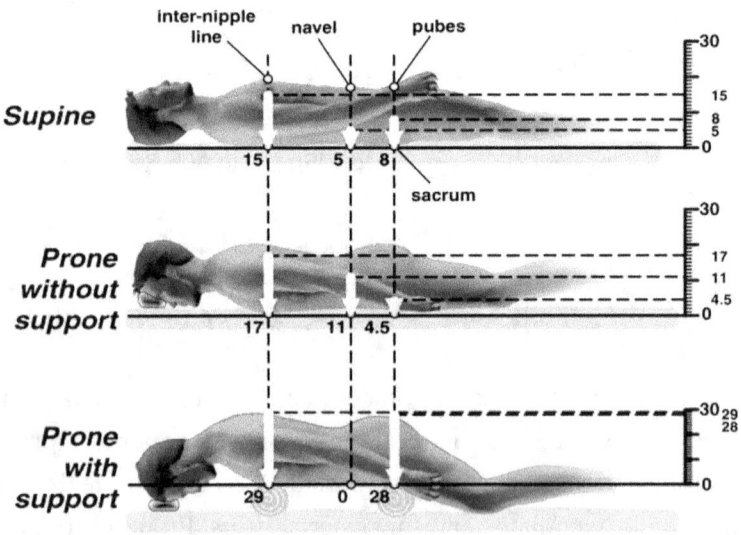

Chiumello et al., 2006 https://www.ncbi.nlm.nih.gov/pubmed/16764731

In order to make the patient comfortable in Prone ventilation position, a pillow can be placed as shown in the picture, since some people have big bellies. The big belly may compress the lungs as a result you may not get the advantage of 20%. How to adjust the pillow can be decided by the comfort level of the patient. Motivate the patient to be in this position for many hours to get the permanent advantage. This is how one can manage the emergency breathing problems.

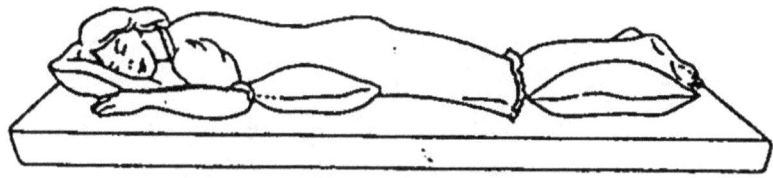

I reiterate that in the hospital set up there are no evidence(s) for oxygen cylinder and mechanical ventilator saving people's lives while there are plenty of evidences in favour of fan being used instead of oxygen cylinder and prone ventilation instead of mechanical ventilator. These evidences clearly state that a set up at home is devoid of side effects and there are increased chances of survival; the chances of mortality are, in fact, reduced. So a patient is safe in the home setting. Don't advise him to go to the hospital since it would worsen his chances of survival.

Managing Uncontrolled Cough

If a person complains of uncontrolled cough, immediately along with the three day Flu diet, start turmeric therapy. Ask the patient to consume a small piece (0.5 gm) of raw/fresh turmeric three times a day- before breakfast, before lunch and before dinner. Normally, we recommend raw/fresh turmeric on the fourth day when the patient is on D.I.P. diet. If the patient does not get relief, double the dose of raw/fresh turmeric i.e. instead of three pieces of raw turmeric, give him raw turmeric pieces six times a day. The cough will be managed in 2-3 days time. Meanwhile, motivate the patient not to lose heart. His problems would subside soon.

Uncontrolled Cough Management

Double the dose of Turmeric
(Six times a day along with the prescribed diet.)

Fever Management

As long as the temperature is ≤ 102° F, there is no need to worry. If the temperature crosses 102° F, go in for cold compress and cold air for 15 minutes. If the patient starts shivering, stop the process. After a gap of half an hour, repeat the process- cold compress and cold air for 15 minutes. If he starts shivering or if the temperature comes down, stop the process. Sometimes the temperature is 103° F -104° F, don't panic. Avoid the intake of anti-pyretic drugs, which may reduce the temperature but not reduce the chances of seizure which may otherwise occur due to increased temperature. There is no evidence that Paracetamol/antipyretic drugs can help a person to live a longer life or it can help to avoid the seizure. Even if temperature gets very high, don't panic because our body has its own homeostasis and will not let the temperature be dangerously high. It knows at what temperature the virus can be killed. So the body has its own mechanism to get rid of the virus. On a safer side, keep providing cold compress and cold air and continue to follow the three day Flu diet.

In my last 12 years of managing the ILI/Flu patients, it has not occurred even once, when the temperature could not be controlled with this strategy.

Vomiting Management

If the patient complains of vomiting, stop his eating and drinking for 4 hours. If need be, simple water or coconut water can be given. Vomiting may not be a comfortable thing but it is not bad either. It is an indication of some infection in the body which the body wants to get rid of. Don't panic. Keep calm. Nobody dies by vomiting. Try to comfort the patient.

Nausea and Weakness

It is seen that many people panic when they feel weak or have nausea. Remember, no one is going to die with weakness and nausea; there won't be any permanent damage either. Comfort the patient by giving him a small piece of fresh ginger 3-4 times a day. Ginger provides strength. If the patient refuses to do so, crush the ginger and boil it in water. Add some lemon and little honey to it. Ask the patient to sip it. He will get strength and energy. Once the temperature subsides, he will get rid of all the problems.

Loose Motions

It has been observed that sometimes patients experience loose motions while following the three step Flu diet. If the loose motions occur more than 6-7 times, then the patient should stop consuming citrus fruit juice (if he is on three step Flu diet) or fruits and salad (if he is on D.I.P. diet) and take only coconut water till loose motions subside or completely stop.

References :

To access the references and videos related to this chapter, go to the link : www.biswaroop.com/nicebook

---

CHAPTER-5

Three Step Flu Diet Study with Government of Maharashtra Covid Centre

Curing Covid-19 in 72 hours!

Specially when the person is a senior citizen with co-morbid condition and presented with severe Pneumonia............... seems to be an impossible feat rather an absurd dream.

However, our consultants and N.I.C.E. practitioners Dr Nilesh Patil and Dr Pallavi Patil could make this impossible.........possible.

The story starts with pursuing the Maharashtra government, Jalgaon Covid-19 centre officials to permit them to treat Covid-19 patients with the 'three step Flu diet'. They got the permission to treat four patients with the condition that the diet needed for the patients would be paid by Dr Nilesh and his team. On July 9, 2020, Dr Nilesh and Dr Pallavi Patil received the patients. Among them two were severely ill with Pneumonia and co-morbid conditions and the rest two were in moderate condition.

By the end of 72 hours of following the three step Flu diet, all of them were relieved of all the Covid-19 symptoms and the three of them tested negative for Covid-19 which includes both the severely ill senior citizens with co-morbid conditions. Please refer to the summary letter issued by the Jalgaon district Covid centre.

Result

After 72 hours of the three step Flu diet,

- 100% of the patients were relieved of all the symptoms.
- 75% of the patients tested negative for Covid-19.

महाराष्ट्र शासन आरोग्य सेवा
ग्रामिण रुग्णालय, पाचोरा, ता.पाचोरा जि.जळगांव

कार्यालय :०२५९६ -२४०१०० कार्यालय
वैद्यकिय अधिक्षक वर्ग-१ यांचे कार्यालय
आरोग्य सेवा
ग्रामिण रुग्णालय पाचोरा
पाचोरा, ता पाचोरा ४२४ २०१.
जा.क्र.ग्रारुपा/ /२०
दिनांक:- / /२०२०

I, Dr. Amit Salunkhe, Medical Superintendent – Rural Hospital Pachora, certifying this report on the request of Dr. Nilesh Patil who had been permitted to undertake COVID -19 patients for Natural Therapy, under the permission granted by District Collector, Jalgaon Mr. Dr. Avinash Dhakne during his visit to COVID Centre ITI Bhadgaon on 7th June 2020.

Maharashtra , District - Jalgaon, Tehsil - Pachora / Bambrud (Govt. Covid-19 Care Centre)
admitted on 9th June
Under Supervision/NICE Team - Dr. Nilesh Patil (MBBS-Ortho Surgeon / Dr. Pallavi Patil (MBBS-Radiologist))

- ❖ 1st Positive Test Report came out – 1 Patient- 8th June/3 Patient-7th June)
- ❖ Handover to NICE Team on 9th June
- ❖ 3 Step Diet (Natural Therapy) started from - 9th to 11th June (3 days)
- ❖ Sample taken for 2nd test on – 12th June
- ❖ 2nd Test Report came out on – 14th June, 2020

S. No	Patient Name	Age/ Gender	First test	Report	P/ N	Second test	Report	P/ N
1.	Bhagabai Nagraj Patil (severe pneumonia with gross xray changes in left lower zone)	F/65	1st June-2020	8th June	P	12 June-20	14th June	N
2.	Prakash Dodu Wani (pneumonia with cardiomegaly)	M/63	5th June-2020	7th June	P	12 June-20	14th June	N
3.	Dipali Shashikant Dhamane	F/19	5th June-2020	7th June	P	12 June-20	14th June	N
4.	Mayuri Shashikant Dhamane	F/23	5th June-2020	7th June	P	12 June-20	14th June	P

Patient No 4- 1) Her Father was expired on 7th June due to Corona Positive
2) She detected Corona Positive on 7th June
3) Her Marriage scheduled on 14th June

Medical Suprintendent Class-I
Rural Hospital,Pachora
Dist.Jalgaon.

Second Study with Maharashtra Government Covid-19 Centre

What happens if the Covid-19 patients follow the three step Flu diet just for 48 hours?

Once again, Dr Nilesh Patil and Dr Pallavi Patil got the permission to treat the Covid-19 patients for 48 hours with the three step Flu diet, but with the condition of bearing the expense of the second Covid-19 test.

This time our N.I.C.E. practitioners received 20 Covid-19 patients for 48 hours (July 2, 2020 to July 3, 2020). The patient with minimum age was of 11 years and the oldest was 85 years of age. Among them, 13 were male and seven were female. On July 14, 2020, the NP swab were taken for Covid-19 test.

Result

- 12 patients tested negative for Covid-19.
- 8 patients tested positive.

Conclusion

60% of the Covid-19 patients could reverse Covid-19 within two days of following the three step Flu diet.

Like Dr. Nilesh & Dr. Pallavi Patil, similar activities are being conducted by the Director General of Police, Shri Hari Narayan Chari Mishra, for the Corona positive policemen in Indore and is able to get Corona negative within 3 to 5 days of prescribing the three step Flu diet. His coverage in the leading newspaper of Indore (Dainik Bhaskar) is testimony of his work.

इंदौर फ्रंट पेज
दैनिक भास्कर
08-06-2020

मंडे पॉजिटिव ■ वीडियो कॉलिंग के जरिये होटल में क्वारेंटाइन पुलिसकर्मियों से खुद बात कर रहे

वियतनाम, कम्बोडिया का इम्युनिटी बढ़ाने वाला डाइट प्लान डीआईजी ने जवानों पर लागू किया, 3 दिन में रिपोर्ट निगेटिव

सुमित ठक्कर | इंदौर

कोरोना संक्रमण की चपेट में आने वाले पुलिसकर्मियों के लिए डीआईजी खुद केयर टेकर बन गए हैं। होटल में क्वारेंटाइन जवानों से वीडियो कॉलिंग के जरिये सेहत का हालचाल जानने के साथ ही उन्होंने विभाग के संक्रमित स्टाफ के लिए इम्युनिटी बढ़ाने वाला एक डाइट प्लान भी तैयार किया है। इस डाइट प्लान के जरिये वे तीन जवानों को ठीक कर चुके हैं। डीआईजी हरिनारायणाचारी मिश्र ने बताया हमने वियतनाम, कंबोडिया और साउथ एशिया के मरीजों पर

भारतीय डॉक्टर्स द्वारा डाइट ट्रीटमेंट को जानकर उसे समझा। इस डाइट में अल्काइन फूड जैसे लिक्विड में नारियल पानी, संतरे का जूस, नींबू और ककड़ी, गाजर को तीन दिन तक तय समयानुसार कोविड पॉजिटिव को दिया गया। इसके सकारात्मक परिणाम सामने आए हैं। जवान नारायण पटेल जो बीते सप्ताह पॉजिटिव निकले थे, तीन दिन उन्हें यह डाइट दी गई। इससे तीन दिन में रिपोर्ट निगेटिव आ गई। तीन और जवानों में तेजी से सुधार हो रहा है। वियतनाम में डॉ. विश्वरूप चौधरी भी इस डाइट ट्रीटमेंट से कई कोविड मरीजों को ठीक कर चुके हैं।

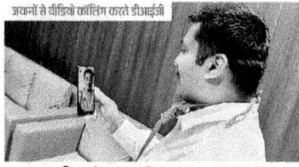
जवानों से वीडियो कॉलिंग करते डीआईजी

कारगर साबित हो सकता है यह डाइट प्लान : डॉक्टर
पल्मोनोलॉजिस्ट डॉ. सलिल भार्गव कहते हैं वे सभी फल और खाने की चीजें जिनमें विटामिन, एंटी ऑक्सिडेंट रहते हैं, वह सब हमारे शरीर की इम्युनिटी बेहतर करते हैं। इसलिए यह डाइट प्लान कारगर साबित हो सकता है।

तीन दिन का डाइट प्लान
पहला दिन : विटामिन सी की लिक्विड डाइट जैसे नींबू पानी, संतरा-मौसंबी का जूस, नारियल पानी दिया जाता है।
दूसरा दिन : अल्काइन फूड में थोड़ा ठोस जैसे गाजर, खीरा (ककड़ी), प्रोटीन के लिए अंडा या अंकुरित अनाज, दूध आदि। दिन में चाय व गर्म पानी में काढ़ा इम्युनिटी बढ़ाने के लिए दिया जाता है।
तीसरा दिन : हार्ड फूड वह भी प्रोटीनयुक्त ही दिया जाता है।

References :

To access the references related to this chapter, go to the link : www.biswaroop.com/nicebook

CHAPTER-6

Build your Own
Super Specialty Hospital @ Home
in Koronakaal

- There is no evidence to show that a mask can protect you from getting infection whereas there is a huge amount of data (as you have seen in the previous chapters) to show that wearing a mask can make you sick.

- There is no evidence and there is no scientific basis that the lockdown can halt or reduce the mortality due to SARS-CoV-2 or any other virus but there are substantial evidences[39] to prove that lockdown resulted in more Corona related deaths and also increased mortality[40] due to the lockdown and social distancing measures. Even WHO has reported[41] in October 2019 that lockdown cannot reduce the mortality from a particular virus.

- All the drugs (anti-HIV/anti-malaria/anti-pyretic/antibiotic) and non-drug medical intervention (ventillator support/plasma therapy) that were experimented on humans in the name of Covid-19 cure without any supporting evidences, however, now we know, have caused more harm and deaths[42].

- There is no evidence either to prove that SARS-CoV-2 is a new virus, a lethal virus and a virus with a high transmission rate. However, I have given enough evidence in the book to prove that it is the other way round.

- With all the evidences and the treatment strategies given in the book, it is safe to conclude that the SARS-CoV-2 is a normal Flu virus and has been there with the mankind for a long time and there is nothing new.

What is new is the mind game- trying to control the population through the weapon of fear, as our psychological consultant Dr Hema Gupta says that the best way to control the human mind is to use the **Walter-Barbe-Raymond Swassing Model** i.e. feeding a fake information, and repeated through all the three senses (auditory, visual and kinesthetic), leading one to believe it to be true and real.

Here the modus operandi is very simple.

Using all the three major senses:

Audio: Repeated warning messages through the caller tune.

Visual: 24 × 7 visual fabricated/fake number of deaths (as I proved in the previous chapters) due to Covid-19 telecasted through television channels.

Kinesthetic: Wearing the mask and sanitizing the hands several times in a day, social distancing etc.

Repeated bombardment of fabricated information several times a day for several days continuously leads to the corrupting of human brain, leading to the disruption of his logical thinking and common sense leading to entering into the mode of slavery.

As a result of the above trickery, the mind of the masses gets corrupted to the extent that they are ready to shell out any amount of money (even Rs 3 lakh to Rs 30 lakh) for a bed in the hospital with the hope of treating Covid-19, which in reality does not exist .

I don't have any doubt that when a shady vaccine will be launched in the name of Covid-19 prevention, all will line up to get one and if the usual and expected side effects of vaccine (including death) occur, then it will be given a new name and will be called a new disease, which co-incidentally arrived at the same time and among the same people who are vaccinated [Do remember every year, on an average 50,000 new cases of vaccine induced Polio occur in India, but they are given a new name AFNPP (Acute Flacid Non Polio Paralysis)][43].

Here the partners to this conspiracy are the pharmaceutical companies and modern medicines using their mouthpiece- the WHO, to create a bizarre rather shocking virus prevention rules. For instance, dead body packed in a plastic bag, to be handed over to the relative, not to be opened and at any moment, not more than two relatives are allowed to be present near the dead body and also minimum one metre distance to be maintained from the dead body[44].

Here if you recall your school text book, you will know that any virus- to multiply and spread in the body is dependent on biochemical energy i.e. adenosine triphosphate (ATP), but once the person is dead, the cells stop making ATP almost immediately after the death hence no possibility of further multiplication of a virus. There may be some virus left which was produced immediately before the death. But in case of SARS-CoV-2, the primary route of transmission is through the droplets expelled while talking, coughing or sneezing. Since the dead bodies cannot breathe, there is no chance of transmission of SARS-CoV-2 through the dead body.

To my understanding, the main cause of creating a special protocol to handle the Covid-19 dead bodies is to cover up the real/true cause of death, which in the majority of cases, is the experimental medication and the lethal untested interventions (plasma therapy). I also fear that prohibiting the kin/relative to see/inspect the dead body will promote an already high margin business of red market (organ trafficking). Reading only one page (page 65) of my book,

Why the Mortality Rate Drops When Doctors Go on Strike?[45] will give you the horrific dark truth of red market.

Now keeping in mind the facts and also the present scenario of the hospitals labelling the non Covid death as Covid death (as discussed in the 1st chapter), it is not advisable to go to the hospital for any reason. Rather it is time to upgrade yourself so that you become your own doctor and let your home be your hospital.

The best way to treat yourself at home is to learn from the revolutionary D.I.P. diet.

From common cold to Cancer,

Depression to Diabetes

This D.I.P. diet can be the fastest, safest and long lasting cure for more than 60 most commonly occurring diseases among humans. Even All India Institute of Ayurveda (under the ministry of Ayush) has conducted clinical trial[46] (TRI/2018/016654, registered on 13/12/2018) for D.I.P. diet, under the guidance of Dr. S.K Gupta (HOD, Department of Shalya Tantra). The research scholar of the trial Dr Monika Sodhe reported a clear cut evidence of benefit in case of the back pain (the primary purpose of the study), the improvement is noted in terms of Thyroid, Blood Sugar, Blood Pressure etc as well.

In fact, in the last 12 years of my clinical practice in India, Vietnam (since 2014) and Malaysia (since 2017), more than 22000 patients from various illnesses have adopted the D.I.P. diet. The time line of reversal of disease based on the feedback of the patients and also my case study reports[47] is as follows:

VIP Diet → D.I.P. Diet	
24hrs to 72hrs	Diabetes
3 days to 1 week	High Blood Pressure, High Cholesterol, Intestinal disorder
1 month	Obesity, Heart Diseases
2 month	Thyroid Disease
6 month	Cancer, Asthma, Arthritis
8 month	Skin Disorder, Kidney dysfunction, Liver disorder

STEPS TO DESIGN YOUR PERSONALIZED D.I.P. DIET:

Step-I

Till 12 noon, eat only fruits of 3 to 4 types including mango, banana, grapes, etc.

Minimum amount to be consumed = Your body weight in kg × 10 = ...gm

For example, a 70 kg person should consume atleast 700 gm of 4 types of fruits before 12 noon.

Step-II

Always eat your lunch/dinner in 2 plates. Plate 1 and Plate 2

Plate 1 should consist of 4 types of vegetables like carrot, tomato, radish and cucumber etc. in raw form.

Lunch/Dinner	
Plate-1 4 types of raw vegetables	**Plate-2** Home cooked vegetarian food

Minimum amount in Plate 1 = Your body weight in kg × 5 = ……….. gm

For example, a 70 kg person should eat at least 350 gm of 4 types of raw vegetables.

Plate 2 should consist of home cooked vegetarian food with negligible salt and oil.

First finish eating from plate 1 in accordance with the above calculation, then take from plate 2 as much as you want. The rules for lunch and dinner are the same; however, you must remember to finish dinner by 7 pm.

Step-III

To Avoid	Snacking
1. Packed food	1. **Soaked nuts:** Your wt(kg) =……gm (For 70kgs person about 70gms of nuts in a day)
2. Refined food	
3. Dairy food/Animal foods	2. **Fruits:** Plenty
4. Nutritional supplements	3. **Coconut water:** As you like
5. Avoid drinking tea/coffee specially before lunch	4. **Hunza Tea:** As you like
	5. **Sprouts:** Your Wt(kg)=…..gm
6. Never eat after 8pm	6. Coconut: As you like
7. NSAID's	7. Sunshine: 45min

You may need to modify and customize the above standard D.I.P. diet based on your symptoms/medical conditions and age. To learn to customize, refer to "Game of Life (GOL)"[48] and you will know that whether you are a third stage Cancer patient or a highly Diabetic- insulin dependent person, the fastest, safest and the long lasting way to cure is at the comfort of your home by using "Food as Medicine".

References :

To access the references and videos related to this chapter, go to the link : www.biswaroop.com/nicebook

SECTION-II

List Of Patients, Who Got Cured Using N.I.C.E Protocol

Below is the list of a few of the 5000+successfully cured patients. We are updating the video testimonials of the patients on continuous basis at www.biswarooop.com/nicebook

Government health agencies may contact us at biswaroop@ biswaroop.com/+91-9313378451 to get access to the complete list of patients with diagnostic documents and related materials.

Patient **Arun Kumar** from *Ludhiana* age **25** yrs reported to N.I.C.E with the symptoms of **Fever, Headache, Body ache/muscle ache, Tiredness** on **28-Jun-20** with co morbidity like **asthma** got cured in **4 days** under the N.I.C.E Care of **Kanishk Amarpuri**

Patient **Jenny Fernandes** from **Kuwait** age **45 yrs** reported to N.I.C.E with the symptoms of **Dry Cough/ Sore throat/Body ache/ muscle ache / Congestion/ Tiredness/Weakness** on **07-Jul-20** got cured in **7 days** under the N.I.C.E Care of **Filda Don**

Patient **Akshay Gorade** from *Mumbai* age **32** yrs reported to N.I.C.E with the symptoms of **Fever, Sore throat, and body ache/ muscle ache** on **26-Jun-20** with co morbidity like **hypertension** got cured in **7 days** under the N.I.C.E Care of **Sudhir Kumar**

Patient **Aakansha** from *New Delhi* age **32** yrs reported to N.I.C.E with the symptoms of **Fever, Dry Cough, Sore throat, Body ache/ muscle ache, Tiredness** on **24-Jun-20** with co morbidity like **hypertension** got cured in **5 days** under the N.I.C.E Care of **Filda Don**

Patient **Narinder Pal Singh** from **Dubai** age **60 yrs** reported to N.I.C.E with the symptoms of **Fever, Dry Cough, Sore throat, Body ache/muscle ache, Tiredness** on **22-Jun-20** got cured in **5 days** under the N.I.C.E Care of **Rupesh Kumar**

Patient **Ajay Arungaikwad** from *Thane* age 27 yrs reported to N.I.C.E with the symptoms of **Fever, Sore throat, Body ache/ muscle ache, Tiredness, breathing difficulty** on 24-Jun-20 with co morbidity like **Heart Disease** got cured in **5 days** under the N.I.C.E Care of **Sounak Das**

Patient **Karshil Shah** from *Ahmedabad* age 12 yrs reported to N.I.C.E with the symptoms of **Fever** on 25-Jun-20 with co morbidity like **hypothyroidism** got cured in **4 days** under the N.I.C.E Care of **Bimal Pal**

Patient **Moin Hussaini** from **Doha** age **49 yrs** reported to N.I.C.E with the symptoms of **Fever, Dry Cough, Sore throat, Headache, Body ache/muscle ache, Tiredness, breathing difficulty** on 28-Jun-20 got cured in **3 days** under the N.I.C.E Care of **Shaikh Warisha Nasim**

Patient **Akbarali Kherdiwala** from **Daman** age **50 yrs** reported to N.I.C.E with the symptoms of **breathing difficulty** on 25-Jun-20 got cured in **4 days** under the N.I.C.E Care of **Satish Kumar Varma Vuppalapati**

Patient **Anisha** from *Pune* age 31 yrs reported to N.I.C.E with the symptom of **breathing difficulty** on 24-Jun-20 with co morbidity like **thyroid** got cured in **6 days** under the N.I.C.E Care of **Dr. C Rajasekhar**

Patient **Mohammad Iqbal** from **Bahrain** sage 42 **yrs** reported to N.I.C.E with the symptoms of Fever, **Tiredness** on 07-Feb-20 got cured in **days** under the N.I.C.E Care of **Rajwinder Kaur**

Patient **Arjun Jagannath Jadhav** from *Kalyan* age 42 yrs reported to N.I.C.E with the symptoms of **Fever, Headache, and body ache/ muscle ache** on 21-Jun-20 with co morbidity like **hypertension** got cured in **6 days** under the N.I.C.E Care of **Sayed Shah**

Patient **Md Shahnawaz** from *Fahaheel* age 45 yrs reported to N.I.C.E with the symptom of **Dry Cough** on 25-Jun-20 with co morbidities like **hypertension, Diabetes, kidney disease** got cured in **4 days** under the N.I.C.E Care of **Kanishk Amarpuri**

Patient **Shaikh Azra** from *Ahmednagar* age **46** yrs reported to N.I.C.E with the symptoms of **Sore throat, breathing difficulty** on **24/Jun-20** with co morbidities like **hypertension, cholesterol** got cured in **3 days** under the N.I.C.E Care of **Ritu Singh**

Patient **Harsh Patel** from *Vapi* age **15** yrs reported to N.I.C.E with the symptoms of **Dry Cough, Headache** on **18-June-20** with co morbidity like **diabetes** got cured in **7 days** under the N.I.C.E Care of **Samir Das**

Patient **Indira Mhatre** from *Dombivli* age **18** yrs reported to N.I.C.E with the symptoms of **breathing difficulty** on **23-June-20** with co morbidity like **Diabetes** got cured in **3 days** under the N.I.C.E Care of **Gopinath Narayanam**

Patient **Biplob Sengupta** from *Siliguri* age **59** yrs reported to N.I.C.E with the symptoms of **Fever, Body ache/muscle ache** on **28-June-20** with co morbidity like **allergic rhinitis** got cured in **6 days** under the N.I.C.E Care of **Sudhir Kumar**

Patient **Vikas** from *Faridabad* age **26** yrs reported to N.I.C.E with the symptoms of **Fever, Dry Cough, Headache, Body ache/muscle ache, Tiredness** on **27-Jun-20** with co morbidities like **Diabetes & kidney disease** got cured in **5 days** under the N.I.C.E Care of **Raj Kishore Kodwani**

Patient **Chander M Rishi** from *Lynnwood* age **73** yrs reported to N.I.C.E with the symptoms of **Sore throat, Headache, Body ache/ muscle ache, Congestion** on **26-Jun-20** with co morbidities like **hypertension, Diabetes** got cured in **4 days** under the N.I.C.E Care of **Bimal Pal**

Patient **Vinod** from *Shimla* age **39** yrs reported to N.I.C.E with the symptoms of **Sore throat, Headache, Body ache/muscle ache, Tiredness** on **12-Jun-20** with co morbidities like **hypertension, Diabetes** got cured in **3 days** under the N.I.C.E Care of **Sunita Dolley**

Patient **Riya Datta** from *Kolkata* age **18** yrs reported to N.I.C.E with the symptoms of **Fever, Headache, Body ache/muscle ache,**

Tiredness, breathing difficulty on **16-Jun-20** with co morbidity like **colitis** got cured in **3 days** under the N.I.C.E Care of **Dharmendra Kumar Pandey**

Patient **Dinanath** from *Dhule* age **42** yrs reported to N.I.C.E with the symptoms of **Dry Cough** on **28-Jun-20** with co morbidity like **hypertension** got cured in **5 days** under the N.I.C.E Care of **Sraban Baraik**

Patient **Sonalben Sodvadiya** from *Surat* age **34** yrs reported to N.I.C.E with the symptoms of **Fever, Sore throat, Headache, Body ache/muscle ache,** on **27-Jun-20** with co morbidity like **hypertension** got cured in **5 days** under the N.I.C.E Care of **Ashok NAdak**

Patient **JK Suri** from *Haryana* age **71** yrs reported to N.I.C.E with the symptoms of **Fever, Dry Cough** on **12-Jun-20** with co morbidity like **Diabetes** got cured in **3 days** under the N.I.C.E Care of **Arun Kumar**

Patient **Vikash Yadav** from *Gurugram* age **18** yrs reported to N.I.C.E with the symptoms of **Fever, Body ache/muscle ache** on **19-Jun-20** with co morbidity like **thyroid** got cured in **4 days** under the N.I.C.E Care of **Biswajit Datta**

Patient **Usha Devi** from *Patna* age **50** yrs reported to N.I.C.E with the symptoms of **Fever, Dry Cough, Body ache/muscle ache, Tiredness** on **2-July-20** with co morbidity like **hypertension** got cured in **6 days** under the N.I.C.E Care of **Dr Seema Arora**

Patient **Puneet Gupta** from *Ghaziabad* age **36** yrs reported to N.I.C.E with the symptom of **Fever** on **26-Jun-20** with co morbidities like **Diabetes and Heart Problem** got cured in **6 days** under the N.I.C.E Care of **Bhagwan Das**

Patient **Dharamveer Singh Gill** from *Dharmkot* age **44** yrs reported to N.I.C.E with the symptoms of **Fever, Body ache/muscle ache, Tiredness** on **19-Jun-20** with co morbidity like **Diabetes** got cured in **5 days** under the N.I.C.E Care of **Sraban Baraik**

Patient **Birendra Sinha** from *Jamui* age **66** yrs reported to N.I.C.E with the symptoms of **Dry Cough, Sore throat, Tiredness** on **9-Jun-20** with co morbidity like **Diabetes** got cured in **4 days** under the N.I.C.E Care of **Chotalia Suresh Chandra**

Patient **Israr Ahmed** from *Dubai* age **35** yrs reported to N.I.C.E with the symptoms of **Fever, Sore Throat, and headache** on 6-Jun-20 with co morbidity like **Epilepsy** got cured in **5 days** under the N.I.C.E Care of **Bhagwan Dass**

Patient **Awdesh** from *Darbhanga* age **36** yrs reported to N.I.C.E with the symptoms of **Fever, Dry Cough** on **27-Jun-20** with co morbidity like **Diabetes** got cured in **7 days** under the N.I.C.E Care of **Nishan Singh Jamwal**

Patient **Aditya** from **Jabalpur** age **20 yrs** reported to N.I.C.E with the symptoms of **Dry Cough, Body ache/muscle ache, Tiredness** on **10-Jun-20 got** cured in **6 days** under the N.I.C.E Care of **Mushtaque Ahmad**

Patient **Ashish Khevji** from **Raichur** age **13 yrs** reported to N.I.C.E with the symptoms of **Fever, Headache** on **25-Jun-20** got cured in **6 days** under the N.I.C.E Care of **Shikha Saxena**

Patient **Jumma Tadavi** from **Jalgaon** age **50 yrs** reported to N.I.C.E with the symptoms of **Fever, Dry Cough, Headache, Body ache/muscleache** on **21-Jun-20** got cured in **4 days** under the N.I.C.E Care of **Bhagwan Dass**

Patient **Mikhael Tirkey** from **Simdega** age **58 yrs** reported to N.I.C.E with the symptoms of **Fever, Headache, and body ache/muscle ache** on **29-Jun-20** got cured in **7 days** under the N.I.C.E Care of **Iqra Shaikh**

Patient **Amit Verma** from **Ghaziabad** age **32 yrs** reported to N.I.C.E with the symptoms of **Fever, Sore throat, Body ache/muscle ache, Tiredness** on **18-Jun-20 got** cured in **3 days** under the N.I.C.E Care of **Dr Seema Arora**

Patient **Anushal Anurag** from **Begusarai** age **28 yrs** reported to N.I.C.E with the symptoms of **Sore throat, Tiredness** on **18-Jun-20** got cured in **6 days** under the N.I.C.E Care of **Samir Das**

Patient **Mamata patra** from **Salipur** age **41 yrs** reported to N.I.C.E with the symptoms of **Sore throat, and breathing difficulty** on **26-Jun-20** got cured in **7 days** under the N.I.C.E Care of **Bimal Pal**

Patient **Arun** from **Dharuhera** age **34 yrs** reported to N.I.C.E with the symptoms of **Fever, Sore throat** on **13-Jun-20 got** cured in **5 days** under the N.I.C.E Care of **Sayed Shah**

Patient **Harneet Kaur** from **Kanpur** age **49 yrs** reported to N.I.C.E with the symptoms of **Fever, Body ache/muscle ache, Tiredness, breathing difficulty** on **16-Jun-20** got cured in **4 days** under the N.I.C.E Care of **Dharmendra Kumar Pandey**

Patient **Mayesha Agarwal** from **Espoo** age **1 yrs** reported to N.I.C.E with the symptoms of **Fever, Body ache/muscle ache** on **15-Jun-20** got cured in **4 days** under the N.I.C.E Care of **Ayan Halder**

Patient **Akarsh** from **Nagpur** age **1.5 yrs** reported to N.I.C.E with the symptoms of **Fever, Tiredness** on **21-Jun-20** got cured in **4 days** under the N.I.C.E Care of **Jasmeet Kaur**

Patient **Vijaya Bhaskar** from **Chengalpattu** age **33 yrs** reported to N.I.C.E with the symptoms of **Congestion** on **09-Jun-20** got cured in **5 days** under the N.I.C.E Care of **Filda Don**

Patient **Yunus** from **Nerul** age **47yrs** reported to N.I.C.E with the symptoms of **Fever, Dry Cough, Sore throat, Tiredness, and breathing difficulty** on **16-Jun-20 got** cured in **4 days** under the N.I.C.E Care of **Shaikh Warisha Nasim**

Patient **Bablu Damai** from **Kharagpur** age **53 yrs** reported to N.I.C.E with the symptoms of **Fever, Body ache/muscle ache, Tiredness** on **27-Jun-20** got cured in **3 days** under the N.I.C.E Care of **Prabin Nanda**

Patient **Pooja Singh** from **Bhopal** age **28 yrs** reported to N.I.C.E with the symptoms of **Fever** on **11-Jun-20** got cured in **6 days** under the N.I.C.E Care of **Kanishk Amarpuri**

Patient **Shinjan Mistry** from **Halisahar** age **8 yrs** reported to N.I.C.E with the symptoms of **Fever, Headache** on **22-Jun-20** got cured in **5 days** under the N.I.C.E Care of **Dr. Barin Kumar**

Patient **Gurbakhash** from **Baghapura** age **46 yrs** reported to N.I.C.E with the symptoms of **Fever, Sore throat, Headache, Body ache/muscle ache** on **20-Jun-20** got cured in **7 days** under the N.I.C.E Care of **Dr Seema Arora**

Patient **Rajesh Burad** from **Malkapur** age **60yrs** reported to N.I.C.E with the symptoms of **Fever, Dry Cough, Sore throat, Congestion, Tiredness** on **23-Jun-20** got cured in **7 days** under the N.I.C.E Care of **Arvind Kumar Plaha**

Patient **Amit Chakraborty** from **Barrackpore** age **40 yrs** reported to N.I.C.E with the symptoms of **Dry Cough, Body ache/muscle ache** on **26-Jun-20** got cured in **3 days** under the N.I.C.E Care of **Nishan Singh Jamwal**

Patient **Sagar Raju Chhapriband** from **Pimpri Chinchwad** age **29 yrs** reported to N.I.C.E with the symptoms of **sore throat, Congestion** on **10-Jun-20** got cured in **4 days** under the N.I.C.E Care of **Mushtaque Ahmad**

Patient **Charan Kaur** from **Moga** age **55 yrs** reported to N.I.C.E with the symptoms of **Fever, Dry Cough, Headache, Body ache/ muscle ache, Congestion, Tiredness, breathing difficulty** on **20-Jun-20** got cured in **5 days** under the N.I.C.E Care of **Shiv Dular**

Patient **Rahil Das** from **Changlang** age **13 yrs** reported to N.I.C.E with the symptom of **Dry Cough** on **18-Jun-20** got cured in **6 days** under the N.I.C.E Care of **Dr. Kishan Pareek**

Patient **Hussain Ghantiwala** from **Secunderabad** age **36 yrs** reported to N.I.C.E with the symptoms of **Body ache/muscle**

ache on **10-Jun-20** got cured in **3 days** under the N.I.C.E Care of **Dr.Manoj Kumar Sharma**

Patient **Chitra Patil** from **Thane** age **47 yrs** reported to N.I.C.E with the symptoms of **Fever, Body ache/muscle ache, Tiredness** on **21-Jun-20** got cured in **7 days** under the N.I.C.E Care of **Bimal Palss**

Patient **Vaishali Jagdale** from **Badlapur** age **38 yrs** reported to N.I.C.E with the symptoms of **Dry Cough, Sore throat, Body ache/muscle ache, Congestion, Tiredness, breathing difficulty** on **26-Jun-20** got cured in **3 days** under the N.I.C.E Care of **Raushan Kumar**

Patient **Sanjana** from **Ulhasnagar** age **43 yrs** reported to N.I.C.E with the symptoms of **Fever, Dry Cough, and Sore throat** on **19-Jun-20** got cured in **4 days** under the N.I.C.E Care of **Kunwar Aryman**

Patient **Shree Daneshwar Mandal** from **Muzaffarpur** age **30 yrs** reported to N.I.C.E with the symptoms of **Sore throat** on **26-Jun-20** got cured in **6 days** under the N.I.C.E Care of **Sanjay Dhaduk**

Patient **Anju Kumar** from **Patna** age **42 yrs** reported to N.I.C.E with the symptoms of **Fever, Headache, and body ache/muscle ache** on **30-Jun-20** got cured in **4 days** under the N.I.C.E Care of **Shiv Dular**

Patient **Dinesh Bhatt** from **Vadodara** age **59 yrs** reported to N.I.C.E with the symptoms of **Fever, Dry Cough, and tiredness** on **18-Jun-20** got cured in **6 days** under the N.I.C.E Care of **Arun Kumar**

Patient **Maujilal Maurya** from **Jaunpur** age **73 yrs** reported to N.I.C.E with the symptoms of and **breathing difficulty** on **24-Jun-20** got cured in **6 days** under the N.I.C.E Care of **Jitendra Kumar Choubey**

Patient **Nazir Jainuddin Hasware** from **Chiplun** age **58 yrs** reported to N.I.C.E with the symptoms of **Fever, Sore throat, Body ache/muscle ache, Tiredness, breathing difficulty** on **03-Jul-20** got cured in **4 days** under the N.I.C.E Care of **Mohammed Rahil Nasim Ahmed**

Patient **Gaurav Kumar** from **Noida** age **17 yrs** reported to N.I.C.E with the symptoms of **Fever, Headache, and tiredness** on **09-Jun-20** got cured in **6 days** under the N.I.C.E Care of **Prabin Nanda**

Patient **Harshita Gupta** from **Rath** age **13 yrs** reported to N.I.C.E with the symptoms of **Fever, Headache, Body ache/muscle ache, Tiredness** on **30-Jun-20** got cured in **5 days** under the N.I.C.E Care of **Sushma Bengani**

Patient **Amol Ahire** from **Nashik** age **26 yrs** reported to N.I.C.E with the symptoms of **Fever, Sore throat, Body ache/muscle ache** on **02-Jul-20** got cured in **6 days** under the N.I.C.E Care of **Dr. Seema Arora**

Patient **Hitendra Singh** from **Gund** age **35 yrs** reported to N.I.C.E with the symptoms of **Body ache/muscle ache, and breathing difficulty** on **18-Jun-20** got cured in **6 days** under the N.I.C.E Care of **Samir Das**

Patient **Imran Khan** from **Sandton** age **35 yrs** reported to N.I.C.E with the symptoms of **Dry Cough, Headache, and body ache/muscle ache** on **30-Jun-20** got cured in **3 days** under the N.I.C.E Care of **Kamlakshi Shahdeo**

Patient **Indtakamal Tiwari** from **Agra** age **27 yrs** reported to N.I.C.E with the symptoms of **Dry Cough** on **28-Jun-20** got cured in **5 days** under the N.I.C.E Care of **Dr. Rajendra Prasad Kumawat**

Patient **Jagdish Sharma** from **Bhiwani** age **33 yrs** reported to N.I.C.E with the symptoms of **Fever, Dry Cough, and body ache/muscle ache** on **16-Jun-20** got cured in **5 days** under the N.I.C.E Care of **Lomash Anand**

Patient **Bhavani Jaiswal** from **Aurangabad** age **23 yrs** reported to N.I.C.E with the symptom of **Sore throat,** on **18-Jun-20** got cured in **3 days** under the N.I.C.E Care of **Dr. Kishan Pareek**

Patient **Renu Devi** from **Jhajjar** age **39 yrs** reported to N.I.C.E with the symptoms of **Dry Cough, Sore throat, Headache, Body ache/ muscle ache, Tiredness** on **11-Jun-20** got cured in **7 days** under the N.I.C.E Care of **Jitendra Kumar Choubey**

Patient **Chetan Chotaliya** from **Rajkot** age **38 yrs** reported to N.I.C.E with the symptoms of **Fever, Dry Cough, Sore throat, Headache, Body ache/muscle ache, Congestion, Tiredness, breathing difficulty** on **30-Jun-20** got cured in **3 days** under the N.I.C.E Care of **Sashapra Chakrawarty**

Patient **Karamjeet Singh** from **Kharar** age **37 yrs** reported to N.I.C.E with the symptoms of **Fever, Sore throat, Tiredness,** on **27-Jun-20** got cured in **4 days** under the N.I.C.E Care of **Kapil Dev Sharma**

Patient **Runu Kar** from **Bhubaneswar** age **49 yrs** reported to N.I.C.E with the symptoms of **Fever, Body ache/muscle ache, Tiredness, breathing difficulty** on **02-Jul-20** got cured in **3 days** under the N.I.C.E Care of **Dr. Kishan Pareek**

Patient **Aman Kesarwani** from **Prayagraj** age **23 yrs** reported to N.I.C.E with the symptoms of **Fever, Headache, Body ache/ muscle ache, Tiredness** on **17-Jun-20** got cured in **6 days** under the N.I.C.E Care of **Sanjay Gupta**

Patient **Shaluta Sandeep Lahane** from **Thane** age **36 yrs** reported to N.I.C.E with the symptoms of **Fever** on **22-Jun-20** got cured in **3 days** under the N.I.C.E Care of **Dr. Barin Kumar Roy**

Patient **Kailash Chandra Pargain** from **Najafgarh** age **24 yrs** reported to N.I.C.E with the symptoms of **Fever, Dry Cough, Sore throat, Headache, Body ache/muscle ache** on **19-Jun-20** got cured in **7 days** under the N.I.C.E Care of **Suresh Kumar Yadav**

Patient **Krishna** from **Lucknow** age **33 yrs** reported to N.I.C.E with the symptoms of **Fever** on **15-Jun-20** got cured in **3 days** under the N.I.C.E Care of **Sourav Bysack**

Patient **Kuldeep Kumar** from **Karnal** age **35 yrs** reported to N.I.C.E with the symptoms of **Body ache/muscle ache** on **11-Jun-20** got cured in **3 days** under the N.I.C.E Care of **Kanishk Amarpuri**

Patient **AK Mishra** from **Bhopal** age **50 yrs** reported to N.I.C.E with the symptoms of **Fever, Body ache/muscle ache, Tiredness** on **29-Jun-20** got cured in **3 days** under the N.I.C.E Care of **Ashish**

Patient **Rajeev Kumar** from **Hapur** age **47 yrs** reported to N.I.C.E with the symptoms of **Fever, Sore throat, Tiredness** on **18-Jun-20** got cured in **3 days** under the N.I.C.E Care of **Kamal Dhawan**

Patient **Kunal** from Madurai **age 23 yrs** reported to N.I.C.E with the symptoms of **Sore throat, Body ache/muscle ache and tiredness** on **27-Jul-20** got cured in **5 days** under the N.I.C.E Care of **Kamak Dhawan**

Patient **Mamta** from **Falna** age **25 yrs** reported to N.I.C.E with the symptoms of **Fever, Headache, Body ache/muscle ache, Tiredness** on **22-Jun-20** got cured in **7 days** under the N.I.C.E Care of **Dr Rajendra Prasad Kumawat**

Patient **Hirabai Renus** from **Airoli** age **65 yrs** reported to N.I.C.E with the symptoms of **Fever, Respiration problem** on **06-Jun-20** got cured in **6 days** under the N.I.C.E Care of **Kodur Venkata Ramana Sastry**

Patient **Mamraj Singh** from **Auraiya** age **40 yrs** reported to N.I.C.E with the symptoms of **Sore throat** on **16-Jun-20** got cured in **5 days** under the N.I.C.E Care of **Sashapra Chakrawarty**

Patient **Manesh Murmu** from **Balurghat** age **39 yrs** reported to N.I.C.E with the symptoms of **Fever, Sore throat** on **16-Jun-20** got cured in **4 days** under the N.I.C.E Care of **Seema Manikkoth**

Patient **Atahagan Manoj Tembhurne** from **Nagpur** age **11 yrs** reported to N.I.C.E with the symptoms of **Fever, Headache,** on **18-**

Jun-20 got cured in **4 days** under the N.I.C.E Care of **Chitra jain**

Patient **Vijay Gupta** from **Jaipur** age **42 yrs** reported to N.I.C.E with the symptoms of **Fever, Body ache/muscle ache** on **09-Jun-20** got cured in **6 days** under the N.I.C.E Care of **Biswajit Datta**

Patient **Dushant Mittal** from **Bathinda** age **26 yrs** reported to N.I.C.E with the symptoms of **Dry Cough, Tiredness** on **26-Jun-20** got cured in **4 days** under the N.I.C.E Care of **Bimal Pal**

Patient **Mousami Goswami** from **Guwahati** age **35 yrs** reported to N.I.C.E with the symptoms of **Fever, Body ache/muscle ache** on **23-Jun-20** got cured in **3 days** under the N.I.C.E Care of **Avinash Popatrao Sabare**

Patient **Lalita Sagar** from **Bharatpur** age **36 yrs** reported to N.I.C.E with the symptoms of **Sore throat, Headache, Body ache/muscle ache** on **18-Jun-20** got cured in **6 days** under the N.I.C.E Care of **Ajeet Singh Foujdar**

Patient **Munish Miglani** from **Hisar** age **22 yrs** reported to N.I.C.E with the symptoms of **breathing difficulty** on **09-Jun-20** got cured in **4 days** under the N.I.C.E Care of **Sona Narang**

Patient **Dilbag Singh** from **Jalandhar** age **26 yrs** reported to N.I.C.E with the symptoms of **Sore throat, Congestion, breathing difficulty** on **28-Jun-20** got cured in **3 days** under the N.I.C.E Care of **Siddharth Jain**

Patient **Narendra Prahlad Naik** from **Jalgaon** age **36 yrs** reported to N.I.C.E with the symptoms of **breathing difficulty** on **02-Jul-20** got cured in **4 days** under the N.I.C.E Care of **Ekta Agarwal**

Patient **Navneet Kumar** from **Narnaul** age **40 yrs** reported to N.I.C.E with the symptoms of **Sore throat, Body ache/muscle ache, breathing difficulty** on **08-Jun-20** got cured in **6 days** under the N.I.C.E Care of **Shikha Saxena**

Patient **Udatbhan** from **Mairwa** age **24 yrs** reported to N.I.C.E with the symptoms of **Sore throat, Body ache/muscle ache, and** tiedness on **24-Jun-20** got cured in **5 days** under the N.I.C.E Care of **Singh Jaiswal**

_____

Patient **Nupur Chaudhary** from **Kanjhawala** age **29 yrs** reported to N.I.C.E with the symptoms of **Sore throat, breathing difficulty** on **02-Jul-20** got cured in **4 days** under the N.I.C.E Care of **Arun Kumar**

_____

Patient **Praveena Abdul Nabi Shaikh** from **Jalna** age **30 yrs** reported to N.I.C.E with the symptoms of **Fever, Body ache/muscle ache** on **23-Jun-20** got cured in **5 days** under the N.I.C.E Care of **Goma Ram**

_____

Patient **Manas Nitin Patil** from **Ambernath** age **6 yrs** reported to N.I.C.E with the symptoms of **Fever, Tiredness** on **20-Jun-20** got cured in **4 days** under the N.I.C.E Care of **Sraban Baraik**

_____

Patient **Pramod Kumar** from **Jabalpur** age **36 yrs** reported to N.I.C.E with the symptoms of **Dry Cough, Sore throat** on **29-Jun-20** got cured in **6 days** under the N.I.C.E Care of **Sudhir Kumar**

_____

Patient **Shashiraj** from **Kurukshetra** age **36 yrs reported** to N.I.C.E with the symptoms of **Fever, Sore throat, Tiredness** on **24-Jun-20** got cured in **7 days** under the N.I.C.E Care of **Ashok N Adak**

_____

Patient **Shiben Das** from **Rangpo** age **31 yrs reported** to N.I.C.E with the symptoms of **Fever, Body ache/muscle ache** on **20-Jun-20** got cured in **6 days** under the N.I.C.E Care of **Nishan Singh Jamwal**

_____

Patient **Sachin Rana** from **Meeranpur** age **24 yrs reported** to N.I.C.E with the symptoms of **Dry Cough, Tiredness, and Sore Throat** on **08-Jun-20** got cured in **5 days** under the N.I.C.E Care of **Brijmohan Yadav**

_____

Patient **Savita Shah** from **Bhiwandi** age **42 yrs reported** to N.I.C.E with the symptom of **Fever** on **18-Jun-20** got cured in **7 days** under the N.I.C.E Care of **Manish Goel**

_____

Patient **Sanjay Sharma** from **Mathabhanga** age **47 yrs** reported to N.I.C.E with the symptoms of **Fever, Dry Cough, Body ache/**

muscle ache, Tiredness on **11-Jun-20** got cured in **3 days** under the N.I.C.E Care of **Suresh Kumar Yadav**

Patient **Roop Singh** from **Ajman** age **28 yrs** reported to N.I.C.E with the symptom of **Fever** on **17-Jun-20 got** cured in **7 days** under the N.I.C.E Care of **Kavitha N Jain**

Patient **Sudhakar Singh Thakur** from **Bilaspur** age **44 yrs** reported to N.I.C.E with the symptom of **Fever** on **20-Jun-20** got cured in **5 days** under the N.I.C.E Care of **Rahul Bansal**

Patient **Suhail Ahmed Shaikh** from **Dammam** age **45 yrs** reported to N.I.C.E with the symptoms of **Sore throat, Tiredness, breathing difficulty** on **22-Jun-20** got cured in **5 days** under the N.I.C.E Care of **Kanishk Amarpuri**

Patient **Suhas Gopal Thorat** from **Panvel** age **40 yrs** reported to N.I.C.E with the symptoms of **Fever, Dry Cough, and sore throat** on **30-Jun-20** got cured in **6 days** under the N.I.C.E Care of **Ashok N Adak**

Patient **Kamlesh Rishi** from **Lynnwood** age **68 yrs** reported to N.I.C.E with the symptoms of **Dry Cough, Sore throat, Headache, Body ache/muscle ache, Congestion** on **26-Jun-20** got cured in **3 days** under the N.I.C.E Care of **Bimal Pal**

Patient **Syed Akheel** from **Abbasiya** age **22 yrs** reported to N.I.C.E with the symptoms of **Fever, Body ache/muscle ache, Tiredness, breathing difficulty** on **28-Jun-20** got cured in **6 days** under the N.I.C.E Care of **Siddharth Jain**

Patient **Sanjay Kumar** from **Kosi kalan** age **47 yrs** reported to N.I.C.E with the symptoms of **Fever, Tiredness,** on **03-Jul-20** got cured in **3 days** under the N.I.C.E Care of **Dr Goutam Paul**

Patient **Saroj Kushwaha** from **Haridwar** age **34** yrs reported to N.I.C.E with the symptom of **Fever** on **17-Jun-20** got cured in **3 days** under the N.I.C.E Care of **Kavitha N Jain**

Patient **Khadka Bahadur Tamang** from **Labor city** age **28 yrs** reported to N.I.C.E with the symptoms of **Fever, Tiredness** on **28-Jun-20** got cured in **7 days** under the N.I.C.E Care of **Shaikh Warisha Nasim**

Patient **Uday Waman Sakurikar** from **Nashik** age **62 yrs** reported to N.I.C.E with the symptoms of **Fever, Body ache/muscle ache, Tiredness** on **21-Jun-20** got cured in **3 days** under the N.I.C.E Care of **Raushan Kumar**

Patient **Ujjal Karmakar** from **Lalgola** age **29 yrs** reported to N.I.C.E with the symptoms of **Dry Cough, Sore throat** on **25-Jun-20** got cured in **6 days** under the N.I.C.E Care of **Sashapra Chakrawarty**

Patient **Meena Jain** from **Bhind** age **53 yrs** reported to N.I.C.E with the symptoms of **Fever, Headache, and Tiredness** on **17-Jun-20** got cured in **6 days** under the N.I.C.E Care of **Siddharth Jain**

Patient **Vishal Pancholi** from **Sahibabad** age **42 yrs** reported to N.I.C.E with the symptoms of **Fever, Headache, Body ache/muscle ache, Tiredness** on **24-Jun-20** got cured in **7 days** under the N.I.C.E Care of **Pradeep chauhan**

Patient **Vijau Mittal** from **Chandigarh** age **64 yrs** reported to N.I.C.E with the symptoms of **Fever, Sore throat** on **26-Jun-20** got cured in **7 days** under the N.I.C.E Care of **Kapil Dev Sharma**

Patient **Kalyan** from **Tezpur** age 35 yrs reported to N.I.C.E with the symptoms of **Dry Cough, Sore throat,** on **25-Jun-20** got cured in **days** under the N.I.C.E Care of **Ashok N Adak**

Patient **Ajay Kumar** from **Astana** age **52 yrs reported** to N.I.C.E with the symptoms of **Headache, Body ache/muscle ache, Tiredness** on **01-Jul-20** got cured in **days** under the N.I.C.E Care of **Dr. Barin Kumar Roy**

Patient **Nazir Jainuddin Hasware** from **Ratnagiri** age **58 yrs** reported to N.I.C.E with the symptoms of **Dry Cough, Sore throat, Headache, Tiredness, Weakness** on **03-Jul-20** got cured in **days** under the N.I.C.E Care of **Dr. Barin Kumar Roy**

Patient **Lewis Fernandes** from **Khaitan, Kuwait** age **12 yrs** reported to N.I.C.E with the symptoms of **Dry Cough, Sore throat ,Bodyache/muscleache,Congestion, Tiredness, Weakness** on 07-Jul-20 got cured in **days** under the N.I.C.E Care of **Savio Paes**

Patient **Irshad** from **Anantapur** age yrs reported to N.I.C.E with the symptoms of **Fever, Dry Cough, and Headache** on 02-Jul-20 got cured in **days** under the N.I.C.E Care of **Nilima N Bhatkar**

Patient **Ankesh** from **Greater Noida** age **27 yrs** reported to N.I.C.E with the symptoms of **Fever, Headache, and Breathing difficulty** on **29-Jun-20** got cured in **days** under the N.I.C.E Care of **Nilima N Bhatkar**

Patient **Umesh Sharma** from **Panvel** age 46yrs reported to N.I.C.E with the symptoms of Fever, **Dry Cough** on 24-Jun-20 **got** cured in **days** under the N.I.C.E Care of **Narendra Singh Patel**

Patient **Luiza Fernandes** from **Kuwait** age 17 yrs reported to N.I.C.E with the suspected symptoms if Influenza/flu on **07-Jul-20** with co - morbidities like **Diabetes and hypertension** got cured in 7 days under the N.I.C.E Care of **Savio Paes.**

Patient **Urbashi Shaw** from **Dehradun** age 31 **yrs** reported to N.I.C.E with the suspected symptoms of Influenza/**flu**/ on **06-Jul-20 got** cured in 7 days under the N.I.C.E Care of **Sounak Das**

Patient **Kashif Patel** from **Latur** age 8 yrs reported to N.I.C.E with the suspected symptoms of Influenza/**flu** on **27-Jun-20** got cured in 7 days under the N.I.C.E Care of **Kamal dhawan**

Patient **Sweta Sekhar Jaipuria** from **Jharsuguda** age 32 yrs reported to N.I.C.E with the suspected symptoms of Influenza/**flu** on **30-Jun-20** got cured in 5 days the N.I.C.E Care of **Mansi Thaker**

Patient Raghu **Thota** from **Al Ain**age 30 yrs reported to N.I.C.E with the suspected symptoms **of Influenza/flu** on **07-Jun-20** got cured in **5** days the N.I.C.E Care of **Daniyal**

Patient Luiza **Fernandes** from **Khaitan, Kuwait** age 17 yrs reported to N.I.C.E with the suspected symptoms of Influenza/**flu** on **07-Jul-20** got cured in **4 days** the N.I.C.E Care of Savio **Paes**

Patient **Bashir Aehamad Maniyar** from **Bijapur** age 59 **yrs** reported to N.I.C.E with the symptoms of Body **ache/muscle ache, Tiredness,** on **29-Jun-20** got cured in **4 days** under the N.I.C.E Care of **Dr. Nidhi Jain** ————————

Patient **Sachin** from **Rohtak** age 24 **yrs** reported to N.I.C.E with the symptoms of Sore **throat, Headache, Body ache/muscle ache, Tiredness, breathing difficulty** on 27-Jun-20 got cured in **7 days** under the N.I.C.E Care of **Gopinath Narayanam**

Patient **Usha Sharma** from **Siliguri** age 28 **yrs** reported to N.I.C.E with the symptoms of Fever, **Dry Cough, Headache, Body ache/muscle ache, Congestion, Tiredness**on 29-Jun-20 got cured in 7 **days** under the N.I.C.E Care of **Manish Goel**

Patient **Ravindra Kumar** from **Forbesganj** age 27 **yrs** reported to N.I.C.E with the symptoms of Fever, **Headache, and Body ache/muscle ache** on 20-Jun-20 got cured in **3 days** under the N.I.C.E Care of **Gopinath Narayanam**

Patient **Mohammad Sarfaraz** from **Riyadh** age 30 **yrs** reported to N.I.C.E with the symptoms of Fever, **Dry Cough, and Sore throat** on 11-Jun-20 got cured in **5 days** under the N.I.C.E Care of **Suresh Kumar Yadav**

Patient **Md Masudal Hoque** from **Damam** age 32 **yrs** reported to N.I.C.E with the symptoms of Fever, **Dry Cough, Sore throat, Headache, Body ache/muscle ache, Congestion, Tiredness, breathing difficulty** on 30-Jun-20 got cured in **4 days** under the N.I.C.E Care of **Utpal Roy**

Patient **Saroj Saini** from **Narela** age 37 **yrs** reported to N.I.C.E with the symptoms of Fever, **Muscle and body aches** on 06-Jun-20 got cured in **6 days** under the N.I.C.E Care of **Nishan Singh Jamwal**

Patient **Satish Nagula** from **Jubail** age 38 **yrs reported** to N.I.C.E with the symptoms of Sore **throat, breathing difficulty** on **26-Jun-20** got cured in **4 days** under the N.I.C.E Care of **Chitra Jain**

Patient **Damanpreet Kaur** from **Banga** age 27 **yrs** reported to N.I.C.E with the symptoms of Fever, **Dry Cough, breathing difficulty** on 19-**Jun-20** got cured in **5 days** under the N.I.C.E Care of **Biswajit Datta**

Patient **Hema** from *New Delhi* age **45** yrs reported to N.I.C.E with the symptoms of **Fever, Dry Cough, Sore throat, Body ache/muscle ache, Tiredness** on **24-Jun-20** with co morbidity like **sleep apnea** got cured in **6 days** under the N.I.C.E Care of **Filda Don**

Patient **Kuldeep** from *West Delhi* age **37** yrs reported to N.I.C.E with the symptoms of **Fever, Headache, and Tiredness** on **21-Jun-20** with co morbidity like **thyroid** got cured in **6 days** under the N.I.C.E Care of **Bimal Pal**

Patient **Mithlesh Jain** from *New Delhi* age **58** yrs reported to N.I.C.E with the symptoms of Fever, **Headache, Body ache/muscle ache, Tiredness** on **22-Jun-20** with co morbidity like **Thyroid** got cured in **7 days**under the N.I.C.E Care of **KimtiLal**

Patient **Amarjit Paswan** from *New Delhi* age **50** yrs reported to N.I.C.E with the symptoms of **Muscle and body aches, Weakness** on **6-Jun-20** with co morbidities like **Sugar, thyroid and cholesterol** got cured in **5 days** under the N.I.C.E Care of **Renu Garg**

Patient **Ajay Kumar** from *New Delhi* age 35 yrs reported to N.I.C.E with the symptoms of **Sore throat, Headache, Tiredness, Breathing difficulty** on **27-Jun-20** with co morbidity like **hypertension** got cured in **3 days** under the N.I.C.E Care of **Chitra Jain**

Patient **Bharti** from *Thane* age 50 yrs reported to N.I.C.E with the symptoms of **Body ache/muscle ache, Tiredness** on **2-July-20** with co morbidity like **spondylitis** got cured in **4 days** under the N.I.C.E Care of **Ashish**

Patient **Mithun Jaju** from *Mumbai* age **40** yrs reported to N.I.C.E with the symptoms of **Sore throat, Body ache/muscle ache,** on **26-**

Jun-20 with co morbidity like **Diabetes** got cured in **5 days** under the N.I.C.E Care of **Ajit Kumar Burnwal**

Patient **Amrita Arya** from *New Delhi* age **26** yrs reported to N.I.C.E with the symptoms of **Fever, Headache, Congestion, and Tiredness** on **21-Jun-20** with co morbidities like **Diabetes, Cirrhosis of liver** Hepatitis E and fluid accumulation in left lung got cured in 6 days under the N.I.C.E Care of **Gaurav Jain**

Patient **Rakesh Shah** from *New Delhi* age **39** yrs reported to N.I.C.E with the symptoms of **Fever, Sore throat** on **16-Jun-20** with co morbidity like **Diabetes Liver disease** got cured in **5 days** under the N.I.C.E Care of **Kamal Dhawan**

Patient **Tahseen Ansari** from *Thane* age **29** yrs reported to N.I.C.E with the symptoms of **Fever, Dry Cough, Sore throat, Tiredness, breathing difficulty** on **24-Jun-20** with co-morbidity like **diabetes** got cured in **7 days** under the N.I.C.E Care of **Atul Jain**

Patient **Sandhya Tukaram Pawar** from *Mumbai* age 47 yrs reported to N.I.C.E with the symptoms of **Dry Cough, Tiredness** on **28-Jun-20** with co morbidity like **hypertension got** cured in **7 days** under the N.I.C.E Care of **Siddharth Jain**

Patient **Neeraj Sharma** from *New Delhi* age **46** yrs reported to N.I.C.E with the symptoms of **Fever, Dry Cough, Headache, Body ache/muscle ache, Tiredness, breathing difficulty** on **27-Jun-20** with co morbidities like **hypertension, Diabetes and fatty liver** got cured in **4 days** under the N.I.C.E Care of **Ekta Agarwal**

Patient **Safura** from *Hyderabad* age **24** yrs reported to N.I.C.E with the symptoms of **Fever, Headache, Body ache/muscle ache, Tiredness** on **25-Jun-20** with co morbidities like **hypertension** got cured in **6 days** under the N.I.C.E Care of **Arpana Madhu Suvarna**

Patient **Brij Mohan** from *New Delhi* age **34** yrs reported to N.I.C.E with the symptoms of **Fever, Dry Cough,Headache,Tiredness** on **10-Jun-20** with comorbidity like **hypertension** got cured in **5days** under the N.I.C.E Care of **Chitra jain**

Patient **Geeta** from *New Delhi* age **22** yrs reported to N.I.C.E with the symptoms of **Fever, Dry Cough, Headache, Tiredness, and breathing difficulty** on **10-June-20** with co morbidity like **hypertension** got cured in **5 days** under the N.I.C.E Care of **Shikha Saxena**

———————————

Patient **Bhawana Tyagi** from *Ahmedabad* age **38**yrs reported to N.I.C.E with the symptoms of **Fever, Body ache/muscle ache, Tiredness** on **13-Jun-20** with co morbidity like **Fatty liver** got cured in **4 days** under the N.I.C.E Care of **Sounak Das**

———————————

Patient **Ajit Yadav** from *New Delhi* age **34** yrs reported to N.I.C.E with the symptoms of **Fever, breathing difficulty** on **11-Jun-20** with co morbidity like **diabetes,** got cured in **4 days** under the N.I.C.E Care of **Biswajit Datta**

———————————

Patient **Dattaramjairamgamre**from *Mumbai Palghar* age **51** yrs reported to N.I.C.E with the symptoms of **Breathing difficulty** on **20-Jun-20** with co morbidity like **Kidney disease** got cured in **5 days** under the N.I.C.E Care of **Sayed Shah**

———————————

Patient **Daya Devendra Pitale** from *Mumbai* age **39** yrs reported to N.I.C.E with the symptoms of **Fever, Dry Cough, Tiredness, Nausea or vomiting, New loss of taste or smell, Muscle and body aches, Headache** on 4-Jun-20 with co morbidity like **Hypertension** got cured in **3 days** under the N.I.C.E Care of **Soumik**

———————————

Patient **Deepak Yadav** from *Kalyan* age **21** yrs reported to N.I.C.E with the symptoms of **Fever, Dry Cough, Headache, Congestion, and breathing difficulty** on **30-Jun-20** with co morbidity like **hypertension** got cured in **7 days** under the N.I.C.E Care of **Ekta Singh**

———————————

Patient **Veena Verma** from *New Delhi* age **60** yrs reported to N.I.C.E with the symptoms of **Fever, Headache, Congestion, and Tiredness** on **18-Jun-20** with co morbidity like **gall bladder stone** got cured in **3 days** under the N.I.C.E Care of **Arun Kumar**

———————————

Patient **Amit Sharma** from New Delhi age 45 yrs reported to N.I.C.E with the symptoms of **Fever, Dry Cough, Sore throat, Headache, Body ache/muscle ache, Congestion, Tiredness, Breathing difficulty** on **24-Jun-20** with co morbidity like **Tuberculosis** got cured in **7 days** under the N.I.C.E Care of **Dr. Kishan Pareek**

Patient **Syed Ali** from *Hyderabad* age **39** yrs reported to N.I.C.E with the symptoms of **Fever, Dry Cough, Sore throat, Body ache/muscle ache, Tiredness** on **28-Jun-20** with co morbidity like **Low blood pressure** got cured in **5 days** under the N.I.C.E Care of **Bhagwan Dass**

Patient **Fayaz Mohammed** from *Hyderabad* age **35** yrs reported to N.I.C.E with the symptoms of **Fever, Body ache/muscle ache, Tiredness** on **9-Jun-20** with co morbidities like **Heart disease and B. P** got cured in **7 days** under the N.I.C.E Care of **Simi Handa**

Patient **Joginder Singh Sabharwal** from *New Delhi* age **68** yrs reported to N.I.C.E with the symptoms of **Fever, Tiredness,** on **14-Jun-20** with co morbidity like **hypertension** got cured in **6 days** under the N.I.C.E Care of **Bimal Pal**

Patient **Yogesh Kumar** from *Delhi* age **35** yrs reported to N.I.C.E with the symptoms of **Dry Cough, Body ache/muscle ache, Tiredness** on **3-July-20** with co morbidities like **hypertension, Diabetes** got cured in **5 days** under the N.I.C.E Care of **Dr. Barin Kumar Roy**

Patient **Gaurav Tyagi** from *Ahmedabad* age **41** yrs reported to N.I.C.E with the symptoms of **Fever, Sore throat, Headache, Body ache/muscle ache, Tiredness** on **10-Jun-20** with co morbidities like **Diabetes** got cured in **6 days** under the N.I.C.E Care of **Kamlakshi Shahdeo**

Patient **Jaskirat Singh** from *Delhi* age **14** yrs reported to N.I.C.E with the symptoms of **Sore throat, Headache** on **9-Jun-20** with co morbidity like **Low Blood Pressure** got cured in **6 days** under the N.I.C.E Care of **Filda Don**

Patient **Riya** from *Surat* age **21** yrs reported to N.I.C.E with the symptoms of **Fever, Body ache/muscle ache, Tiredness** on 24-Jun-20 with co morbidity like **hypertension** got cured in **3 days** under the N.I.C.E Care of **Karan Shetty**

Patient **Suhasini Pawar** from *Kalyan* age 49 yrs reported to N.I.C.E with the symptoms of **Fever, Headache, and Body ache/muscle ache** on 2-July-20 with co morbidity like **Kidney stones** got cured in **7 days** under the N.I.C.E Care of **Arun Kumar**

Patient **Gulam Rafeeq Ahmed** from *Hyderabad* age 34 yrs reported to N.I.C.E with the symptoms of **Dry Cough, Tiredness, and breathing difficulty** on 26-Jun-20 got cured in **4 days** under the N.I.C.E Care of **Ajit Kumar Burnwal**

Patient **Ankit** from *Delhi* age **24** yrs reported to N.I.C.E with the symptoms of **Dry Cough** on **12-Jun-20** with co morbidity like **heart disease got** cured in **7 days** under the N.I.C.E Care of **Sunita Dolley**

Patient **Harish Kumar Rohilla** from *New Delhi* age **35** yrs reported to N.I.C.E with the symptom of **tiredness, bodyache,** on 21-Jun-20 with co morbidity like **Diabetes** got cured in **6 days** under the N.I.C.E Care of **Suresh Kumar Yadav**

Patient **Gurdeep Singh** from *Delhi* age 63 yrs reported to N.I.C.E with the symptoms of **Fever, Dry Cough, Body ache/muscle ache, Congestion, Tiredness, breathing difficulty** on 9-Jun-20 with co morbidity like **kidney failure** got cured in **6 days** under the N.I.C.E Care of **Jasmeet Kaur**

Patient **Rekha Sharma** from *Gurugram* age **38** yrs reported to N.I.C.E with the symptoms of **Fever, Dry Cough, Sore throat, Headache, Body ache/muscle ache, Congestion, Tiredness** on 21-Jun-20 with co morbidity like **hypertension** got cured in **7 days** under the N.I.C.E Care of **Siddharth Jain**

Patient **Vinod** from *Shimla* age 34 yrs reported to N.I.C.E with the symptoms of **Sore throat, breathing difficulty** on 29-Jun-20 with co morbidity like **asthma** got cured in **5 days** under the N.I.C.E Care of **Dr. C Rajasekhar**

Patient **Ismail, D.** from *Hyderabad* age **52** yrs reported to N.I.C.E with the symptoms of **Sore throat** on **28-Jun-20** with co morbidity like **hypertension** got cured in **5 days** under the N.I.C.E Care of **Sraban Baraik**

Patient **Santpriya Swami** from *Ahmedabad* age **55** yrs reported to N.I.C.E with the symptoms of **Fever, Dry Cough, Headache, and Body ache/muscle ache** on **29-Jun-20** with co morbidity like **hypertension got** cured in **7 days** under the N.I.C.E Care of **Rupesh Kumar**

Patient **Kavita Ajay Athavale** from *Kalyan* age **40** yrs reported to N.I.C.E with the symptoms of **Fever, Dry Cough, Headache, and Tiredness** on **26-Jun-20** with co morbiditiy like **Diabetes** got cured in **4 days** under the N.I.C.E Care of **Suresh Kumar Yadav**

Patient **Harinder Mohan** from *Delhi* age **57** yrs reported to N.I.C.E with the symptoms of **Fever, Sore throat, Body ache/muscle ache, Congestion, Tiredness** on **18-Jun-20** with co morbidity like **hypertension** got cured in **4 days** under the N.I.C.E Care of **Kamal Dhawan**

Patient **Satish Kumar** from *New Delhi* age **55** yrs reported to N.I.C.E with the symptoms of **breathing difficulty** on **11-Jun-20** with co morbidity like **heart disease** got cured in **4 days** under the N.I.C.E Care of **Jitendra Kumar Choubey**

Patient Kiran **Kadam from *Dombivli*** age **26** yrs reported to N.I.C.E with the symptoms of **Fever, Congestion** on **26-Jun-20** with co morbidity like **heart disease** got cured in **7 days** under the N.I.C.E Care of **Kapil Dev Sharma**

Patient **Kalpana** from *Delhi* age **33** yrs reported to N.I.C.E with the symptoms of **Fever, Dry Cough, Sore throat, Headache, Body ache/muscle ache, Congestion, Tiredness, Bbreathing difficulty** on **21-Jun-20** with co morbidity like **Thyroid** got cured in **5 days** under the N.I.C.E Care of **Ignore**

Patient **Kamal Kumar** from *New Delhi* age **39** yrs reported to N.I.C.E with the symptom of **Fever on 15-Jun-20** with co morbidity like **Diabetes** got cured in **4 days** under the N.I.C.E Care of **Ashish**

Patient **Sanjeev Kapur** from *New Delhi* age **55** yrs reported to N.I.C.E with the symptoms of **Fever, Dry Cough, Sore throat, Headache, Body ache/muscle ache** on **24-Jun-2020** with co morbidity like **Heart Disease** got cured in **3 days** under the N.I.C.E Care of **Pradeep Chauhan**

Patient **Vijay Daga** from *Mumbai* age **50** yrs reported to N.I.C.E with the symptoms of **Fever, Body ache/muscle ache, Congestion** on **20-Jun-20** with co morbidities like **hypertension, Diabetes** got cured in **3 days** under the N.I.C.E Care of **Dr Rajendra Prasad Kumawat**

Patient **Aditya Ramdev Jaiswar** from *Mumbai* age **26** yrs reported to N.I.C.E with the symptom of **Dry Cough** on **11-Jun-20** with co morbidity like **asthma from birth** got cured in **4 days** under the N.I.C.E Care of **Kanishk Amarpuri**

Patient **Dileep Kumar** from **New Delhi** age **28 yrs** reported to N.I.C.E with the symptoms of Fever, **Dry Cough, Sore throat, Headache, Body ache/muscle ache, Congestion, Tiredness** on **16-Jun-20** got cured in **4 days** under the N.I.C.E Care of **Kamal Dhawan**

Patient **Ravi Kumar** from **New Delhi** age **26 yrs** reported to N.I.C.E with the symptoms of **Fever, Sore throat, Body ache/muscle ache, Tiredness,** on **17-Jun-20** got cured in **4 days** under the N.I.C.E Care of **Prabin Nanda**

Patient **Anil Patel** from **Mumbai** age **48 yrs** reported to N.I.C.E with the symptoms of **Fever, Dry Cough, Headache, Congestion, breathing difficulty** on **11-Jun-20** got cured in **6 days** under the N.I.C.E Care of **Sounak Das**

Patient **Abhishek Jain** from **New Delhi** age **29 yrs** reported to N.I.C.E with the symptoms of **Fever, Headache, Body ache/muscle ache, Tiredness** on **12-Jun-20** got cured in **5 days** under the N.I.C.E Care of **Bimal Pal**

Patient **Huda** from **Hyderabad** age **23 yrs** reported to N.I.C.E with the symptoms of **Fever, Headache, Body ache/muscle ache, Tiredness** on **13-Jun-20 got** cured in **6 days** under the N.I.C.E Care of **Dr.Manoj Kumar Sharma**

Patient **Abhijit Adhikary** from **Kolkata** age **60 yrs** reported to N.I.C.E with the symptoms of **Fever, Dry Cough, Sore throat, Tiredness** on **26-Jun-20** got cured in **5 days** under the N.I.C.E Care of **Prabin Nanda**

Patient **Aditya Jain** from **Faridabad** age **28 yrs** reported to N.I.C.E with the symptom of **Tiredness** on **18-Jun-20** got cured in **5 days** under the N.I.C.E Care of **Lomash Anand**

Patient **Rahul jain** from **New Delhi** age **33 yrs reported** to N.I.C.E with the symptoms of **Fever, Headache, Body ache/muscle ache, Tiredness** on **22-Jun-20 got** cured in **4 days** under the N.I.C.E Care of **Kimti Lal**

Patient **Mohamed Waheed Uddin** from **Hyderabad** age **54 yrs reported** to N.I.C.E with the symptoms of **Fever, Dry Cough, and breathing difficulty** on **01-Jul-20** got cured in **7 days** under the N.I.C.E Care of **Nishan Singh Jamwal**

Patient **Anup Agarwal** from **Hyderabad** age **33 yrs** reported to N.I.C.E with the symptoms of **Breathlessness & stomach pain** on **07-Jun-20** got cured in **6 days** under the N.I.C.E Care of **Biswajit Datta**

Patient **Ajay Kumar**from **New Delhi** age **52 yrs** reported to N.I.C.E with the symptoms of **Headache, Body ache/muscle ache, Tiredness** on **01-Jul-20 got** cured in **4 days** under the N.I.C.E Care of **Dr. Barin Kumar Roy**

Patient **Rakhi** from **New Delhi** age **31 yrs** reported to N.I.C.E with the symptoms of **Dry Cough** on **01-Jul-20** got cured in **3 days** under the N.I.C.E Care of **Filda Don**

Patient **Ajay Chawla** from **New Delhi** age **63 yrs** reported to N.I.C.E with the symptoms of **Fever, Body ache/muscle ache, Tiredness** on **13-Jun-20** got cured in **4 days** under the N.I.C.E Care of **Rahul Bansal**

Patient **J.K.Sachdeva** from **New Delhi** age **80 yrs** reported to N.I.C.E with the symptoms of **Fever, Tiredness** on **29-Jun-20** got cured in **3 days** under the N.I.C.E Care of **Ritu Singh**

Patient **Ajay** from **Faridabad** age **36 yrs** reported to N.I.C.E with the symptoms of **Fever, Headache, and Body ache/muscle ache** on **12-Jun-20** got cured in **4 days** under the N.I.C.E Care of **Renu Garg**

Patient **Ajay Kumar Shaw** from **Kolkata** age **49 yrs** reported to N.I.C.E with the symptoms of **Fever, Dry Cough, and Body ache/ muscle ache** on **16-Jun-20 got** cured in **6 days** under the N.I.C.E Care of **Dharmendra Kumar Pandey**

Patient **Ajay** from **Faridabad** age **26 yrs** reported to N.I.C.E with the symptoms of **Sore throat, Body ache/muscle ache** on **09-Jun-20** got cured in **7 days** under the N.I.C.E Care of **Kanishk Amarpuris**

Patient **Dhanush Santosh Thombare** from **Mumbai** age **1 yrs** reported to N.I.C.E with the symptoms of **Fever, Dry Cough** on **10-Jun-20** got cured in **7 days** under the N.I.C.E Care of **Suman Chauhan**

Patient **Anis Fatima** from **Hyderabad** age **44 yrs** reported to N.I.C.E with the symptoms of **Fever, Headache, Body ache/muscle ache, Tiredness** on **24-Jun-20** got cured in **6 days** under the N.I.C.E Care of **Atul Jain**

Patient **Alok Ranjan** from **Kolkata** age **28 yrs** reported to N.I.C.E with the symptoms of **Fever, Headache, and Tiredness** on **03-Jul-20** got cured in **7 days** under the N.I.C.E Care of **Dr Goutam Paul**

Patient **Ansuya Siddhapura** from **Mumbai** age **68 yrs** reported to N.I.C.E with the symptoms of **Fever, Breathing difficulty** on **30-Jun-20** got cured in **5 days** under the N.I.C.E Care of **Shiv Dular**

Patient **Amit Babar** from **Ahmedabad** age **27 yrs** reported to N.I.C.E with the symptom of **Fever** on **02-Jul-20** got cured in **6 days** under the N.I.C.E Care of **Dr. Kishan Pareek**

Patient **Amena Kausar** from **Hyderabad** age **60 yrs** reported to N.I.C.E with the symptoms of **Headache, Body ache/muscleache** on **01-Jul-20 got** cured in **11 days** under the N.I.C.E Care of **Dr. Barin Kumar Roy**

Patient **Aniket** from **New Delhi** age **29yrs** reported to N.I.C.E with the symptoms of **Fever, Dry Cough, Sore throat, Body ache/ muscle ache, Tiredness, Breathing difficulty** on **20-Jun-20** got cured in **5 days** under the N.I.C.E Care of **Sayed Shah**

Patient **Deepak** from **New Delhi** age **27 yrs** reported to N.I.C.E with the symptoms of **Fever, Headache, Body ache/muscle ache, Congestion** on **16-Jun-20** got cured in **6 days** under the N.I.C.E Care of **Shaikh Warisha Nasim**

Patient **Kumar Gereja** from **Pune** age **50 yrs** reported to N.I.C.E with the symptoms of **Fever, Dry Cough, and Tiredness** on **23-Jun-20** got cured in **7 days** under the N.I.C.E Care of **Dharmendra Kumar Pandey**

Patient **Anshu Pandey** from **Gurugram** age **34 yrs** reported to N.I.C.E with the symptoms of **Fever, Dry Cough, Sore throat, Congestion, Breathing difficulty** on **17-Jun-20** got cured in **3 days** under the N.I.C.E Care of **Chotalia Suresh Chandra**

Patient **Anup Singh** from **New delhi** age **44 yrs** reported to N.I.C.E with the symptoms of **Fever, Dry Cough, Headache, Body ache/ muscle ache, Tiredness, Breathing difficulty** on **12-Jun-20** got cured in **5 days** under the N.I.C.E Care of **Deepti V Helgaonkar**

Patient **Anupam Sharma** from **New Delhi** age **23 yrs** reported to

N.I.C.E with the symptoms of **Dry Cough, Headache, and Body ache/muscle ache, breathing difficulty** on **26-Jun-20** got cured in **6 days** under the N.I.C.E Care of **Sanjay Dhaduk**

Patient **Annu Sharma** from **New Delhi** age **43 yrs** reported to N.I.C.E with the symptoms of **Fever, Dry Cough** on **29-Jun-20** got cured in **3 days** under the N.I.C.E Care of **Raushan Kumar**

Patient **Pramod Jain** from **New Delhi** age **53 yrs** reported to N.I.C.E with the symptoms of **Dry Cough, Body ache/muscle ache, Tiredness** on **12-Jun-20** got cured in **5 days** under the N.I.C.E Care of **Sunita Dolley**

Patient **Neelam Arneja** from **New Delhi** age **56 yrs** reported to N.I.C.E with the symptoms of **Fever, Sore throat, Headache, Body ache/muscle ache** on **09-Jun-20 got** cured in **4 days** under the N.I.C.E Care of **Simi Handa**

Patient **Neelam** from **New Delhi** age **56 yrs** reported to N.I.C.E with the symptoms of **Fever, Sore throat, Headache, Body ache/ muscle ache** on **06-Sep-20** got cured in **3 days** under the N.I.C.E Care of **Simi Handa**

Patient **Arpita Chougale** from **Pune** age **37 yrs** reported to N.I.C.E with the symptoms of **Fever, Body ache/muscle ache, Tiredness** on **16-Jun-20** got cured in **4 days** under the N.I.C.E Care of **Dr. S Bengani**

Patient **Tejas Kutal** from **Pune** age **15 yrs** reported to N.I.C.E with the symptom of **Headache** on **7-Jun-20** got cured in **7 days** under the N.I.C.E Care of **Sayed Shah**

Patient **Aryan Luthra** from **New Delhi** age **17 yrs** reported to N.I.C.E with the symptoms of **Fever, Dry Cough, Headache, Body ache/muscle ache, Tiredness** on **26-Jun-20** got cured in **5 days** under the N.I.C.E Care of **Filda Don**

Patient **Ashok Agarwal** from **Mumbai** age **47yrs** reported to N.I.C.E with the symptoms of **Fever, Dry Cough, Sore throat, Body ache/ muscle ache, Congestion, Tiredness, breathing difficulty** on **02-**

Jul-20 got cured in **4 days** under the N.I.C.E Care of **Dharmendra Kumar Pandey**

Patient **Ashwani Taneja** from **Faridabad** age **11 yrs** reported to N.I.C.E with the symptoms of **Fever, Headache, Body ache/muscle ache, Tiredness** on **21-Jun-20** got cured in **5 days** under the N.I.C.E Care of **Rahul Bansal**

Patient **Atul Thokale** from **Kalyan** age **38 yrs** reported to N.I.C.E with the symptoms of **Fever, Dry Cough, Headache, Body ache/muscle ache** on **16-Jun-20** got cured in **4 days** under the N.I.C.E Care of **Avinash Popatrao Sabare**

Patient **Avinash Narayan Dhokare** from **Dombivali** age **33 yrs** reported to N.I.C.E with the symptoms of **Fever, Dry Cough, Headache, Body ache/muscleache** on **27-Jun-20 got** cured in **4 days** under the N.I.C.E Care of **Kapil Dev Sharma**

Patient **Mohammed Azharuddin** from **Hyderabad** age **25 yrs** reported to N.I.C.E with the symptoms of **Dry Cough, Sore throat, Tiredness** on **09-Jun-20** got cured in **6 days** under the N.I.C.E Care of **Najabhai Bhagvanbhai Chauhan**

Patient **Bharat Salvi** from **Kalyan** age **33 yrs** reported to N.I.C.E with the symptoms of **Fever, Dry Cough, Headache, Body ache/muscle ache, Tiredness** on **22-Jun-20** got cured in **7 days** under the N.I.C.E Care of **Suresh Venkatrao Garad**

Patient **Bhavya Aggarwal** from **New Delhi** age **24 yrs** reported to N.I.C.E with the symptoms of **Sore throat, Tiredness** on **09-Jun-20** got cured in **5 days** under the N.I.C.E Care of **Rahul Bansal Roy**

Patient **Sourabh** from **Bengaluru** age **42 yrs** reported to N.I.C.E with the symptom of **Fever** on **30-Jun-20** got cured in **3 days** under the N.I.C.E Care of **Arpana Madhu Suvarna**

Patient **British Yadav** from **Mumbai** age **32 yrs** reported to N.I.C.E with the symptoms of **Fever, Sore throat, Headache, Body ache/muscle ache, Congestion** on **13-Jun-20** got cured in **5 days** under the N.I.C.E Care of **Utpal Roy**

Patient **Akash Jindal** from **Faridabad** age **30 yrs** reported to N.I.C.E with the symptoms of **Fever, Sore throat, Body ache/muscle ache, Tiredness, breathing difficulty** on 22-Jun-20 **got** cured in **6 days** under the N.I.C.E Care of **Dr Rajendra Prasad Kumawat**

Patient **Bimla** from **New Delhi** age **50 yrs** reported to N.I.C.E with the symptoms of **Fever, Dry Cough, Headache, and Tiredness** on 13-Jun-20 got cured in **5 days** under the N.I.C.E Care of **Chitra jain**

Patient **Chanda** from **New Delhi** age **38 yrs** reported to N.I.C.E with the symptoms of **Fever, Body ache/muscle ache** on 21-Jun-20 got cured in **4 days** under the N.I.C.E Care of **Sounak Das**

Patient **Vijendra Kumar Chaubey** from **Ahemdabad** age **34yrs reported** to N.I.C.E with the symptoms of **Fever, Headache, and Tiredness** on 19-Jun-20 got cured in **4 days** under the N.I.C.E Care of **Neelima Chatterjee**

Patient **Srilatha** from **Bengaluru** age **38 yrs** reported to N.I.C.E with the symptoms of **Fever, Body ache/muscle ache, Tiredness** on 16-Jun-20 got cured in **6 days** under the N.I.C.E are of **Dr. Kishan Pareek**

Patient **Amarjeet Singh** from **New Delhi** age **34yrs** reported to N.I.C.E with the symptoms of **Nausea or Vomiting, Headache** on 06-Jun-20 got cured in **7 days** under the N.I.C.E Care of **Ashish**

Patient **Rajveer Kahlon** from **Pune** age **10 yrs** reported to N.I.C.E with the symptoms of **Headache, Congestion** on 28-Jun-20 got cured in **3 days** under the N.I.C.E Care of **Nirmala Pandey**

Patient **Datta Shedge** from **Navi Mumbai** age **35 yrs** reported to N.I.C.E with the symptoms of **Fever, Dry Cough, breathing difficulty** on 21-Jun-20 got cured in **3 days** under the N.I.C.E Care of **Chitra jain**

Patient **Preeti Dokania** from **New Delhi** age **47 yrs** reported to N.I.C.E with the symptoms of **Fever, Sore throat, Body ache/**

muscle ache on 19-Jun-20 got cured in **5 days** under the N.I.C.E Care of **Ashish**

Patient **Deepak Jangir** from **New Delhi** age **21 yrs** reported to N.I.C.E with the symptoms of **Dry Cough** on **26-Jun-20** got cured in **7 days** under the N.I.C.E Care of **Gaurav Jain**

Patient **Deepak Nagarkoti** from **New Delhi** age **33 yrs** reported to N.I.C.E with the symptoms of **Fever, Dry Cough, Headache, Body ache/muscle ache, Congestion, Tiredness, breathing difficulty** on **01-Jul-20** got cured in **6 days** under the N.I.C.E Care of **Rahul Bansal**

Patient **Vidya Devi** from **New Delhi** age **70 yrs** reported to N.I.C.E with the symptoms of Fever, **Dry Cough, Tiredness, Sore Throat, Congestion, New loss of taste or smell, Muscle and body aches,** on **06-Jun-20** got cured in **3 days** under the N.I.C.E Care of **Suresh Kumar Yadav**

Patient **Jeyarajan Iyappan** from **Thane** age **41 yrs** reported to N.I.C.E with the symptoms of **Fever, Body ache/muscle ache, Tiredness** on **09-Jun-20** got cured in **4 days** under the N.I.C.E Care of **Ajit Kumar Burnwal**

Patient **Sandhya** from **Bengaluru** age **45 yrs** reported to N.I.C.E with the symptoms of **Fever, Dry Cough, and Tiredness on 30-Jun-20** got cured in **4 days** under the N.I.C.E Care of **Arun Kumar**

Patient **Dil Kumari Pandey** from **Mumbai** age **35 yrs** reported to N.I.C.E with the symptoms of **Fever, Dry Cough, Headache, Body ache/muscle ache, Tiredness** on **25-Jun-20** got cured in **4 days** under the N.I.C.E Care of **Manish Arya**

Patient **Dipesh Jain** from **Secundrabad** age **30 yrs** reported to N.I.C.E with the symptoms of **Fever, Headache** on **02-Jul-20** got cured in **3 days** under the N.I.C.E Care of **Sushma Bengani**

Patient **Snehal Thakker** from **Ahmedabad** age **29 yrs** reported to N.I.C.E with the symptoms of **Fever, Dry Cough** on **07-Jun-20** got cured in **5 days** under the N.I.C.E Care of **Manish Goel**

Patient **Ishkant Sharma** from **New Delhi** age **15 yrs** reported to N.I.C.E with the symptoms of **Fever, Headache** on **15-Jun-20** got cured in **4 days** under the N.I.C.E Care of **Ayan Halder**

Patient **Ram Khatri** from **New Delhi** age **38 yrs** reported to N.I.C.E with the symptom of **Fever** on **09-Jun-20** got cured in **5 days** under the N.I.C.E Care of **Siddharth Jain**

Patient **Manan Oberoi** from **Gurugram** age **21 yrs** reported to N.I.C.E with the symptoms of **Fever, Headache** on **29-Jun-20** got cured in **4 days** under the N.I.C.E Care of **Samir Das**

Patient **Diksha** from **New Delhi** age **24 yrs reported** to N.I.C.E with the symptoms of **Fever, Sore throat, Tiredness** on **19-Jun-20** got cured in **3 days** under the N.I.C.E Care of **Rupesh Kumar**

Patient **Fareeha** from **Hyderabad** age **14 yrs reported** to N.I.C.E with the symptom of **Dry Cough** on **03-Jul-20** got cured in **3 days** under the N.I.C.E Care of **Dr. Barin Kumar Roy**

Patient **Syed Arshad Ali** from **Hyderabad** age **38 yrs reported** to N.I.C.E with the symptoms of **Dry Cough, Headache, and breathing difficulty** on **30-Jun-20** got cured in **6 days** under the N.I.C.E Care of **Arpana Madhu Suvarna**

Patient **Zainab** from **Hyderabad** age **23 yrs reported** to N.I.C.E with the symptoms of **Fever, Dry Cough, Headache, Breathing difficulty** on **30-Jun-20** got cured in **5 days** under the N.I.C.E Care of **Shiv Dular**

Patient **Farzana** from **Delhi** age **30 yrs reported** to N.I.C.E with the symptoms of **Fever, Sore throat, Tiredness** on **26-Jun-20 got** cured in **4 days** under the N.I.C.E Care of **Gopinath Narayanam**

Patient **Mohammed Fazil Siddiqui** from **Hyderabad** age **50 yrs reported** to N.I.C.E with the symptoms of **Fever, Body ache/ muscle ache, Tiredness** on **26-Jun-20** got cured in **3 days** under the N.I.C.E Care of **Ekta singh**

Patient **Divyanshu Gupta** from **New Delhi** age **15 yrs reported** to N.I.C.E with the symptoms of **Dry Cough, Sore throat, Body ache/muscle ache, Congestion, Tiredness, breathing difficulty** on **29-Jun-20** got cured in **4 days** under the N.I.C.E Care of **Bhagwan Dass**

Patient **Kirti Gambhir** from **Mumbai** age **38 yrs reported** to N.I.C.E with the symptoms of **Sore throat, Congestion** on **28-Jun-20** got cured in **6 days** under the N.I.C.E Care of **Nirmala Pandey**

Patient **Ginni Khurana** from **New Delhi** age **68yrs reported** to N.I.C.E with the symptoms of **fever, Dry Cough,** on **16-Jun-20** got cured in **4 days** under the N.I.C.E Care of **Seema Manikkoth**

Patient **Charanjeet Kaur** from **Delhi** age **49 yrs reported** to N.I.C.E with the symptoms of **Fever, Dry Cough, Sore throat, Headache, Body ache/muscleache** on **09-Jun-20** got cured in **5 days** under the N.I.C.E Care of **Filda Don**

Patient **Gurjeet Singh** from **Delhi** age **23 yrs reported** to N.I.C.E with the symptoms of **Fever, Sore throat, Headache, Body ache/muscle ache** on **09-Jun-20** got cured in **4 days** under the N.I.C.E Care of **Sona Narang**

Patient **Gaurav Singh** from **Noida** age **32 yrs reported** to N.I.C.E with the symptoms of **Fever, Dry Cough, and Tiredness** on **30-Jun-20** got cured in **7 days** under the N.I.C.E Care of **Arpana Madhu Suvarna**

Patient **Tarun Chauhan** from **New Delhi** age **29 yrs reported** to N.I.C.E with the symptoms of **Fever, Body ache/muscle ache, Tiredness** on **16-Jun-20** got cured in **3 days** under the N.I.C.E Care of **Hemraj Jagannath Saner**

Patient **Gulabrao** from **Vasai West** age **64 yrs reported** to N.I.C.E with the symptom of **Dry Cough** on **22-Jun-20** got cured in **4 days** under the N.I.C.E Care of **Nishu Sandhya**

Patient **Atma Ram** from **Gurugram** age **75 yrs reported** to N.I.C.E with the symptoms of **Fever, Tiredness** on **28-Jun-20** got cured in **4 days** under the N.I.C.E Care of **Ritu Singh**

Patient **Rashmi Gupta** from **Delhi** age **40 yrs reported** to N.I.C.E with the symptoms of **Fever, Dry Cough, and Sore throat** on 30-**Jun-20** got cured in **7 days** under the N.I.C.E Care of Avinash **Popatrao Sabare**

Patient **Gurudev** from **New Delhi** age **17 yrs reported** to N.I.C.E with the symptoms of **Tiredness, Muscle and body ache** on 05-**Jun-20** got cured in **4 days** under the N.I.C.E Care of **Suresh Chotalia**

Patient **Prakash Chugria** from **Ulhasnagar** age **58 yrs reported** to N.I.C.E with the symptoms of **Fever, Dry Cough, and Tiredness** on 26-**Jun-20** got cured in **6 days** under the N.I.C.E Care of **Sudhir Kumar**

Patient **Shailesh Gangaram hate** from **Mumbai** age **38 yrs reported** to N.I.C.E with the symptoms of **Fever, Sore throat, Body ache/ muscle ache, Tiredness** on 20-**Jun-20** got cured in **7 days** under the N.I.C.E Care of **Nishan Singh Jamwal**

Patient **Narender Kumar** from **Gurugram** age 38 **yrs reported** to N.I.C.E with the symptoms of **Fever, Sore throat, Body ache/ muscle ache, Tiredness** on 19-**Jun-20** got cured in **7 days** under the N.I.C.E Care of **Sraban Baraik**

Patient **Harsh Gupta** from **Delhi** age 21 **yrs reported** to N.I.C.E with the symptoms of **Fever, Dry Cough, Sore throat, Headache, breathing difficulty** on 22-**Jun-20** got cured in **6 days** under the N.I.C.E Care of **Dr. Rajendra Prasad Kumawat**

Patient **Himanshu Raheja** from delhi age **34 yrs reported** to N.I.C.E with the symptoms of **Sore throat, Breathing difficulty** on 11-**Jun-20** got cured in **4 days** under the N.I.C.E Care of **Shruti Sharma**

Patient **Mohammed Sadiq** from **Hyderabad** age 40 **yrs reported** to N.I.C.E with the symptoms of **Fever, Headache, Body ache/ muscle ache, Tiredness** on 02-**Jul-20** got cured in **5 days** under the N.I.C.E Care of **Shaikh Warisha Nasim**

Patient **Devaki B. Rewadkar** from **Mumbai** age 61 **yrs reported** to N.I.C.E with the symptoms of **Fever, Headache, Body ache/ muscle ache, Tiredness** on 30-Jun-20 got cured in **4 days** under the N.I.C.E Care of **Arun Kumar**

Patient **Piyush** from **Gurugram** age 33 **yrs reported** to N.I.C.E with the symptoms of **breathing difficulty** on 26-Jun-20 got cured in **6 days** under the N.I.C.E Care of **Nishan Singh Jamwal**

Patient I**slam Ahmed** from **Delhi** age 28 **yrs reported** to N.I.C.E with the symptoms of **Fever, Sore throat, Headache, Body ache/ muscle ache, Tiredness, breathing difficulty** on 21-Jun-20 got cured in **7 days** under the N.I.C.E Care of **Sounak Das**

Patient **Anil Devani** from **Ahmedabad** age 47 **yrs reported** to N.I.C.E with the symptoms of **Fever, breathing difficulty** on 09-Jun-20 got cured in **6 days** under the N.I.C.E Care of **Hemraj Saner**

Patient **Mohd. Jahangir** from **Hyderabad** age 25 **yrs reported** to N.I.C.E with the symptoms of **Dry Cough, Headache, Body ache/ muscle ache** on 29-Jun-20 got cured in **6 days** under the N.I.C.E Care of **Sudhir Kumar**

Patient **Deepika Jain** from **Delhi** age 41 **yrs reported** to N.I.C.E with the symptoms of **Fever, Sore throat, Headache, Body ache/ muscle ache, Tiredness** on 01-Jul-20 got cured in **3 days** under the N.I.C.E Care of **Rajeev Kumar**

Patient **Vaibhav Jain** from **SURAT** age 24 **yrs reported** to N.I.C.E with the symptoms of **Dry Cough, Headache, Body ache/muscle ache, Tiredness** on 26-Jun-20 got cured in **7 days** under the N.I.C.E Care of **Rahul Bansal**

Patient **Jasdeep Kaur** from **New Delhi** age 42 **yrs reported** to N.I.C.E with the symptoms of **Fever, Headache** on 22-Jun-20 got cured in **3 days** under the N.I.C.E Care of **Bimal Pal**

Patient **Jaspal Singh** from **Delhi** age **44 yrs reported** to N.I.C.E with the symptoms of **Fever, Dry Cough, Congestion, Tiredness** on **13-Jun-20** got cured in **5 days** under the N.I.C.E Care of **Gaurav Jain**

Patient **Dhan Singh** from **Noida** age 57 **yrs reported** to N.I.C.E with the symptoms of **Tiredness** on 18-**Jun-20** got cured in **7 days** under the N.I.C.E Care of **Goma Ram**

Patient **Vinod Chagdev Kadam** from **Mumbai** age 40 **yrs reported** to N.I.C.E with the symptoms of **Fever, Headache, and Body ache/ muscle ache** on 26-**Jun-20** got cured in **4 days** under the N.I.C.E Care of **Dr. Rajendra Prasad Kumawat**

Patient **Savitaben Narenbhai Pandav** from **SURAT** age 48 **yrs reported** to N.I.C.E with the symptoms of **Fever, Dry Cough, and Tiredness** on 26-**Jun-20** got cured in **7 days** under the N.I.C.E Care of **Goma Ram**

Patient **Anuradha Ramsagar Singh** from **Mumbai** age **49 yrs reported** to N.I.C.E with the symptoms of **Dry Cough** on 20-**Jun-20** got cured in **3 days** under the N.I.C.E Care of **Brijmohan Yadav**

Patient **Sanjay Kapoor** from **Delhi** age 57 **yrs reported** to N.I.C.E with the symptoms of **Fever, Dry Cough, Sore throat, Headache, Body ache/muscle ache, Tiredness** on 29-**Jun-20** got cured in **4 days** under the N.I.C.E Care of **Gopinath Narayanam**

Patient **Ketkee** from **Pune** age 33 **yrs reported** to N.I.C.E with the symptoms of **Sore throat, Congestion** on 29-**Jun-20** got cured in **5 days** under the N.I.C.E Care of **Sudhir Kumar**

Patient **Devender** from **Delhi** age 41 **yrs reported** to N.I.C.E with the symptoms of **Fever, Dry Cough** on 24-**Jun-20** got cured in **3 days** under the N.I.C.E Care of **Ananta Kumar Panda**

Patient **Arvind Kumar** from **Delhi** age 45 **yrs reported** to N.I.C.E with the symptoms of **Fever, Dry Cough, Body ache/muscle ache, Tiredness, No Symptoms/ Asymptomatic** on 21-**Jun-20** got cured in **5 days** under the N.I.C.E Care of **Biswajit Datta**

Patient **Kunal** from **Madurai** age **23 yrs reported** to N.I.C.E with the symptoms of **Sore throat, Body ache/muscle ache, Tiredness** on **27-Jun-20** got cured in **5 days** under the N.I.C.E Care of **Kamal Dhawan**

Patient **Kundan Kumar Singh** from **New Delhi** age 28 yrs **reported** to N.I.C.E with the symptoms of **Fever, Dry Cough** on 25-Jun-20 got cured in **3 days** under the N.I.C.E Care of **Arun Kumar**

Patient **Karan Arora** from **New Delhi** age 36 yrs **reported** to N.I.C.E with the symptoms of **Fever, Sore throat, Body ache/muscle ache, Tiredness** on 09-Jun-20 got cured in **5 days** under the N.I.C.E Care of **Rahul Bansal**

Patient **Laxman Gupta** from **Bengaluru** age 22 **yrs reported** to N.I.C.E with the symptoms of **Fever, Body ache/muscle ache** on 14-**Jun-20** got cured in **4 days** under the N.I.C.E Care of **Bimal Pal**

Patient **Lalit Kumar Singhi** from **Kolkata** age 53 **yrs reported** to N.I.C.E with the symptoms of **Fever, Dry Cough, and Sore throat** on 21-**Jun-20** got cured in **3 days** under the N.I.C.E Care of **Kapil Dev Sharma**

Patient **M B Azad** from **New Delhi** age 55 yrs **reported** to N.I.C.E with the symptoms of **Fever, Dry Cough, Body ache/muscle ache, Tiredness** on 11-**Jun-20** got cured in **5 days** under sthe N.I.C.E Care of **Dr Rajendra Prasad Kumawat**

Patient **Manik Lal Gupta** from **Lucknow** age 47 **yrs reported** to N.I.C.E with the symptoms of **Fever, Sore throat, Tiredness, breathing difficulty** on 09-**Jun-20** got cured in **7 days** under the N.I.C.E Care of **Poonam Arora**

Patient **Madhusuudan** from **Pune** age 62 **yrs reported** to N.I.C.E with the symptoms of Fever on 07-**Jun-20** got cured in **3 days** under the N.I.C.E Care of **Ishank Kumar Varshney**

Patient **Raman Kumar Jain** from **Hyderabad** age 42 **yrs reported** to N.I.C.E with the symptoms of **Headache, Body ache/muscle ache** on 27-**Jun-20** got cured in **3 days** under the N.I.C.E Care of **Suresh Kumar Yadav**

Patient **Pratiksha Tiwari** from **Bengaluru** age 30 **yrs reported** to N.I.C.E with the symptoms of **Fever, Body ache/muscle ache** on 16-**Jun-20** got cured in **3 days** under the N.I.C.E Care of **Dr. Kishan Pareek**

Patient **Mr Bal Mukund Sharma** from **New Delhi** age 87 **yrs reported** to N.I.C.E with the symptoms of **Fever, Dry Cough, Sore throat, Headache, Body ache/muscle ache, Congestion, Tiredness, breathing difficulty** on 28-Jun-20 got cured in **7 days** under the N.I.C.E Care of **Karan Shetty**

Patient **Kulwant Singh** from **New Delhi** age 30 **yrs reported** to N.I.C.E with the symptoms of **Fever, Sore throat, Headache, Body ache/muscle ache, Tiredness** on 10-Jun-20 got cured in **4 days** under the N.I.C.E Care of **Karan Shetty**

Patient **Atul Kumar Chhabra** from **New Delhi** age 35 **yrs reported** to N.I.C.E with the symptoms of **Sore throat, Headache, Tiredness** on 09-**Jun-20** got cured in **3 days** under the N.I.C.E Care of **Pratik Anand**

Patient **Saanvi Budharapu** from **Mumbai** age 32 **yrs reported** to N.I.C.E with the symptoms of **Body ache/muscle ache, Tiredness** on 10-**Jun-20** got cured in **6 days** under the N.I.C.E Care of **Punyaa**

Patient **Ramesh Jha** from **Navi Mumbai** age 55 **yrs reported** to N.I.C.E with the symptoms of **Fever, Headache, Body ache/ muscle ache** on 18-Jun-20 got cured in **3 days** under the N.I.C.E Care of **Chitra jain**

Patient **Rafat** from **Hyderabad** age 35 **yrs reported** to N.I.C.E with the symptoms of **Fever, Dry Cough, Headache, Congestion, and Tiredness** on 24-Jun-20 got cured in **6 days** under the N.I.C.E Care of **Atul Jain**

Patient **Amit Mandlik** from **Mumbai** age 33 **yrs reported** to N.I.C.E with the symptoms of **Fever** on 21-**Jun-20** got cured in 3 **days** under the N.I.C.E Care of **Deepti V Helgaonkar**

Patient **Surender Lal** from **New Delhi** age 66 **yrs reported** to

N.I.C.E with the symptoms of **Fever, Sore throat, Body ache/ muscle ache** on **14-Jun-20** got cured in **6 days** under the N.I.C.E Care of **Brajakishore Sinha**

Patient **Manender Singh** from **New delhi** age 34 **yrs reported** to N.I.C.E with the symptoms of **Sore throat, Tiredness** on **25-Jun-20** got cured in **5 days** under the N.I.C.E Care of **Reena Thakur**

Patient **Ramniklal Maru** from **Thane** age **75 yrs reported** to N.I.C.E with the symptoms of **Fever** on **26-Jun-20** got cured in **6 days** under the N.I.C.E Care of **Manish Goel**

Patient **Udit Mathur** from **Delhi** age 30 **yrs reported** to N.I.C.E with the symptoms of **Fever, Headache, and Body ache/muscle ache** on **19-Jun-20** got cured in **3 days** under the N.I.C.E Care of **Sudhir Kumar**

Patient **Mayank** from **Delhi** age 25 **yrs reported** to N.I.C.E with the symptoms of **Body ache/muscle ache, Tiredness** on **18-Jun-20** got cured in **7 days** under the N.I.C.E Care of **Dr. Kishan Pareek**

Patient **Kamlesh** from **Delhi** age **50 yrs reported** to N.I.C.E with the symptoms of **Fever, Dry Cough, Sore throat, Headache, Body ache/muscle ache, Congestion, Tiredness, breathing difficulty** on **09-Jun-20** got cured in **6 days** under the N.I.C.E Care of **Preethi Katariya**

Patient **Meenu** from **Delhi** age 26 **yrs reported** to N.I.C.E with the symptoms of **Fever, Headache** on **20-Jun-20** got cured in **3 days** under the N.I.C.E Care of **Goma Ram**

Patient **Meharwan Singh** from **Greater Noida** age 50 **yrs reported** to N.I.C.E with the symptoms of **Fever, Dry Cough, Sore throat, Body ache/muscle ache, Congestion, Tiredness, breathing difficulty** on **08-Jun-20** got cured in **3 days** under the N.I.C.E Care of **Ekta**

Patient **Kames Mehto** from **Khoda colony** age **29 yrs reported** to N.I.C.E with the symptoms of **Headache, Body ache/muscle ache,**

Tiredness on 26-Jun-20 got cured in **5 days** under the N.I.C.E Care of **Girish Banvi**

Patient **Mahalingam K** from **Bengaluru** age 68 **yrs reported** to N.I.C.E with the symptoms of **Fever, Dry Cough, and Tiredness** on 29-**Jun-20** got cured in **3 days** under the N.I.C.E Care of **Rupesh Kumar**

Patient **Khaja Moinuddin** from **Hyderabad** age 41 **yrs reported** to N.I.C.E with the symptoms of **Sore throat, Body ache/muscle ache, Congestion, Tiredness** on 27-**Jun-20** got cured in **3 days** under the N.I.C.E Care of **Suresh Kumar Yadav**

Patient **Suman** from **Palam Colony** age 25 **yrs reported** to N.I.C.E with the symptoms of **Headache, Tiredness** on 10-**Jun-20** got cured in **4 days** under the N.I.C.E Care of **Mushtaque Ahmad**

Patient **Ranjit Kaur** from **Delhi** age 66 yrs reported to N.I.C.E with the symptoms of **Tiredness** on 18-**Jun-20** got cured in **7 days** under the N.I.C.E Care of **Lomash Anand**

Patient **Manish Singh Rajput** from **Delhi** age 24 **yrs reported** to N.I.C.E with the symptoms of **Fever, Dry Cough, and Headache** on 26-**Jun-20** got cured in **7 days** under the N.I.C.E Care of **Goma Ram**

Patient **Hema** from **Delhi** age 26 **yrs reported** to N.I.C.E with the symptoms of **Fever, Headache, and Body ache/muscle ache** on 17-**Jun-20** got cured in **5 days** under the N.I.C.E Care of **Sashapra Chakrawarty**

Ghatge from **Mumbai** age 48 **yrs reported** to N.I.C.E with the symptoms of **Fever, Dry Cough, Headache, Body ache/muscle ache, Tiredness** on 29-**Jun-20** got cured in **4 days** under the N.I.C.E Care of **Gopinath Narayanam**

Patient **Sunil Gupta** from **Delhi** age 54 **yrs reported** to N.I.C.E with the symptoms of **Fever, Congestion, and Tiredness** on 09-**Jun-20** got cured in **7 days** under the N.I.C.E Care of **Sanjay Dhaduk**

Patient **Syed Reza** from **Bengaluru** age 22 **yrs reported** to N.I.C.E with the symptoms of **Fever, Sore throat, Headache, Tiredness** on 24-**Jun-20** got cured in **3 days** under the N.I.C.E Care of **Filda Don**

Patient **Rajendri** from **Delhi** age 57 **yrs reported** to N.I.C.E with the symptoms of **Fever, Dry Cough, Sore throat, Body ache/ muscle ache, Tiredness** on 27-**Jun-20** got cured in **4 days** under the N.I.C.E Care of **Prabin Nanda**

Patient **Rahul Rathod** from **Ahmedabad** age 30 **yrs reported** to N.I.C.E with the symptoms of **Dry Cough** on 09-**Jun-20** got cured in **7 days** under the N.I.C.E Care of **Rishu Garg**

Patient **Udaybhan** from **Mairwa** age 24 **yrs reported** to N.I.C.E with the symptoms of **Body ache/muscle ache, Tiredness** on 24-**Jun-20** got cured in **5 days** under the N.I.C.E Care sof **Nishan Singh Jamwal**

Patient **Nisha Kadam** from Thane age **36 yrs reported** to N.I.C.E with the symptoms of **Fever, Sore throat, Headache, Body ache/ muscle ache** on 22-**Jun-20** got cured in **6 days** under the N.I.C.E Care of **Atish R. Jaiswal**

Patient **Vinay** from **Delhi** age 43 **yrs reported** to N.I.C.E with the symptoms of **Sore throat** on 30-**Jun-20** got cured in **4 days** under the N.I.C.E Care of **Goma Ram**

Patient **Sujit** from **Faridabad** age 35 **yrs reported** to N.I.C.E with the symptoms of **Fever, Body ache/muscle ache, Congestion, Tiredness** on 02-**Jul-20** got cured in **7 days** under the N.I.C.E Care of **Arun Kumar**

Patient **Santosh Rani** from **New Delhi** age 52 **yrs reported** to N.I.C.E with the symptoms of **Body ache/muscle ache, Tiredness** on 08-**Jun-20** got cured in **3 days** under the N.I.C.E Care of **Shikha Saxena**

Patient **Poonam Kumari** from **Faridabad** age 28 **yrs reported** to N.I.C.E with the symptoms of **Fever, Dry Cough, Headache, Body ache/muscle ache, Congestion, Tiredness** on 21-**Jun-20** got cured in **3 days** under the N.I.C.E Care of **Kodur Venkata Ramana Sastry**

Patient **Aryan** from **Delhi** age 18 **yrs reported** to N.I.C.E with the symptoms of **Fever, Dry Cough, Sore throat, breathing difficulty** on 17-**Jun-20** got cured in **7 days** under the N.I.C.E Care of **Kavitha N Jain**

Patient **Pardeep Kumar Yadav** from **Gurugram** age 41 **yrs reported** to N.I.C.E with the symptoms of **Sore throat, breathing difficulty** on 02-**Jul-20** got cured in **6 days** under the N.I.C.E Care of **Ashish**

Patient **Paresh Shah** from **Pune** age 36 **yrs reported** to N.I.C.E with the symptoms of **Sore throat** on 27-**Jun-20** got cured in **5 days** under the N.I.C.E Care of **Suresh Kumar Yadav**

Patient **Parvez** from **Faridabad** age 29 **yrs reported** to N.I.C.E with the symptoms of **Sore throat, Body ache/muscle ache, Tiredness** on 09-**Jun-20** got cured in **6 days** under the N.I.C.E Care of **Pratik Anand**

Patient **Parveen** from **Delhi** age 37 **yrs reported** to N.I.C.E with the symptoms of **Fever, Dry Cough, and Tiredness** on 24-**Jun-20** got cured in **6 days** under the N.I.C.E Care of **Madhuri Anand Kinikar**

Patient **Pavan Jain Kala** from **Hyderabad** age 57 **yrs reported** to N.I.C.E with the symptoms of **Fever, Dry Cough, Headache** on 26-**Jun-20** got cured in **6 days** under the N.I.C.E Care of **Gopinath Narayanam**

Patient **Pawan Kumar** from **Delhi** age 22 **yrs reported** to N.I.C.E with the symptoms of **Dry Cough** on 16-**Jun-20** got cured in **7 days** under the N.I.C.E Care of **Dr. Ekta Agarwal**

Patient **Vazirchand Ailani** from **Thane** age 80 **yrs reported** to N.I.C.E with the symptoms of **Fever, Tiredness** on 23-**Jun-20** got cured in **6 days** under the N.I.C.E Care of **Samir Das**

Patient **Srushti R. Pisat** from **Thane** age 19 **yrs reported** to N.I.C.E with the symptoms of **Sore throat** on 29-**Jun-20** got cured in **7 days** under the N.I.C.E Care of **Milesh Sahare**

Patient **Piyush Gaur** from **New Delhi** age 27 **yrs reported** to N.I.C.E with the symptoms of **Fever, Sore throat, Congestion, breathing difficulty** on 25-**Jun-20** got cured in **6 days** under the N.I.C.E Care of **Sounak Das**

Patient **Dalip Kumar** from **Delhi** age 43 **yrs reported** to N.I.C.E with the symptoms of **Fever, Headache** on 26-**Jun-20** got cured in **4 days** under the N.I.C.E Care of **Filda Don**

Patient **Poonam Sangle** from **Lake Forest** age 20 **yrs reported** to N.I.C.E with the symptoms of **Fever, Dry Cough, Sore throat, Body ache/muscle ache, Congestion, Tiredness** on 10-**Jun-20** got cured in **3 days** under the N.I.C.E Care of **Pratik Anand**

Patient **Pradeep Vishwakarma** from **Mumbai** age 22 **yrs reported** to N.I.C.E with the symptoms of **Fever** on 18-**Jun-20** got cured in **6 days** under the N.I.C.E Care of **Bhagwan Dass**

Patient **Manas Sundar nayak** from **Gurugram** age 37 **yrs reported** to N.I.C.E with the symptoms of **Fever, Dry Cough, Sore throat, Congestion** on 15-**Jun-20** got cured in **5 days** under the N.I.C.E Care of **Sourav Bysack**

Patient **Vikas Dubey** from **Delhi** age **33 yrs reported** to N.I.C.E with the symptoms of **Fever, Dry Cough, loss of taste or smell, Muscle and body aches** on **07-Jun-20** got cured in **4 days** under the N.I.C.E Care of **Dr Rajendra Prasad Kumawat**

Patient **Prashant from Delhi** age 33 **yrs reported** to N.I.C.E with the symptoms of **Fever, Sore throat, Body ache/muscle ache** on 20-**Jun-20** got cured in **3 days** under the N.I.C.E Care of **Sanjay Dhaduk**

Patient **Pratik Eknath Gharat** from **Navi Mumbai** age 28 **yrs reported** to N.I.C.E with the symptoms of **Fever, Dry Cough, Headache, Body ache/muscle ache** on 27-**Jun-20** got cured in **5 days** under the N.I.C.E Care of **Dilbag Singh**

Patient **Praveen Kumar** from **Aurangabad** age 32 **yrs reported** to N.I.C.E with the symptoms of **Fever, Tiredness** on 01-**Jul-20** got cured in **6 days** under the N.I.C.E Care of **Raushan Kumar**

Patient **Praveen Kumar** from **Aurangabad** age 27 **yrs reported** to N.I.C.E with the symptoms of **Dry Cough, Sore throat** on 25-**Jun-20** got cured in **5 days** under the N.I.C.E Care of **Kamlakshi Shahdeo** ————————

Patient **Pravesh Rahangdale** from **Nagpur** age **38 yrs reported** to N.I.C.E with the symptoms of **Fever** on **07-Jun-20** got cured in **5 days** under the N.I.C.E Care of **Manish Goel**

Patient **Priyanka Pathak** from **Govindpuri** age 1 **yrs reported** to N.I.C.E with the symptoms of **Fever, Sore throat, Body ache/ muscle ache, Tiredness** on 17-**Jun-20** got cured in **7 days** under the N.I.C.E Care of **Avinash Popatrao Sabare**

Patient **Vishal Sehgal** from **Delhi** age 29 **yrs reported** to N.I.C.E with the symptoms of **Dry Cough, Headache, and Tiredness** on 25-**Jun-20** got cured in **3 days** under the N.I.C.E Care of **Sashapra Chakrawarty** ————————

Patient **Pritpal Singh** from **Delhi** age **30 yrs reported** to N.I.C.E with the symptoms of **Fever, Dry Cough, Sore throat** on **16-Jun-20** got cured in **6 days** under the N.I.C.E Care of **Kamal Dhawan**

Patient **Puja Gupta** from **Kolkata** age **27 yrs reported** to N.I.C.E with the symptoms of **Fever, Headache, Body ache/muscle ache, Tiredness** on **26-Jun-20** got cured in **4 days** under the N.I.C.E Care of **Jasmeet Kaur** ————————

Patient **Pushpalata Rao** from **Kalyan** age 51 **yrs reported** to N.I.C.E with the symptoms of **Fever, Dry Cough, Headache, Body ache/ muscle ache, Tiredness** on 27-**Jun-20** got cured in **6 days** under the N.I.C.E Care of **Ajit Kumar Burnwal**

Patient **Ved Parkash Verma** from **New Delhi** age 57 **yrs reported** to N.I.C.E with the symptoms of **Fever** on 20-**Jun-20** got cured in **3 days** under the N.I.C.E Care of **Shubhangi Godse**

Patient **Pawan Wadhwa** from **Delhi** age 58 **yrs reported** to N.I.C.E with the symptoms of **Fever, Dry Cough, Sore throat, Body ache/**

muscle ache, **Tiredness** on 11-**Jun-20** got cured in **7 days** under the N.I.C.E Care of **Raushan Kumar**

Patient **Naresh chandok** from **New delhi** age **55 yrs reported** to N.I.C.E with the symptoms of **Fever, Body ache/muscle ache** on 12-**Jun-20** got cured in **4 days** under the N.I.C.E Care of **Ekta Singh**

Patient **Seema Wadhwa** from **Delhi** age **19 yrs reported** to N.I.C.E with the symptoms of **Fever, Sore throat, Headache, Tiredness** on 19-**Jun-20** got cured in **3 days** under the N.I.C.E Care of **Rupesh Kumar**

Patient **Seema Bhatia** from **Delhi** age **45 yrs reported** to N.I.C.E with the symptoms of Fever, **Dry Cough, Sore throat, Headache, Body ache/muscle ache, Congestion, Tiredness, breathing difficulty** on 08-**Jun-20** got cured in **3 days** under the N.I.C.E Care of **Rupesh Kumar**

Patient **Subhan** from **Hyderabad** age **20 yrs reported** to N.I.C.E with the symptoms of **Fever, Sore throat, Body ache/muscle ache** on 02-**Jul-20** got cured in **6 days** under the N.I.C.E Care of **Ajeet Singh**

Patient **Shallu** from **Delhi** age **32 yrs reported** to N.I.C.E with the symptoms of **Fever** on 16-**Jun-20** got cured in **3 days** under the N.I.C.E Care of **Kamal Dhawan**

Patient **Shambhoo** from **Delhi** age **36 yrs reported** to N.I.C.E with the symptom of **breathing difficulty** on 30-**Jun-20** got cured in **4 days** under the N.I.C.E Care of **Mushtaque Ahmad**

Patient **Zahir Qureshi** from **Kalyan** age **64 yrs reported** to N.I.C.E with the symptoms of **Fever, Sore throat, Headache, Body ache/ muscle ache, Tiredness** on 26-**Jun-20** got cured in **3 days** under the N.I.C.E Care of **Jasmeet Kaur**

Patient **Humera sultana** from **Hyderabad** age **34 yrs reported** to N.I.C.E with the symptoms of **Fever, Headache, Body ache/muscle** ache, **Tiredness** on 26-Jun-20 **got** cured in **4 days** under the N.I.C.E Care of **Brijmohan Yadav**

Patient **Shashi Kalaker** from **Hyderabad** age **41 yrs reported** to N.I.C.E with the symptoms of **Dry Cough, Sore throat** on 26-Jun-20 got cured in **4 days** under the N.I.C.E Care of **Nishan Singh Jamwal**

Patient **Shivam Vishwakarma** from **West Delhi** age **21 yrs reported** to N.I.C.E with the symptoms of Fever, **Headache, Body ache/muscle ache, Tiredness** on 30-Jun-20 got cured in **4 days** under the N.I.C.E Care of **Ashok N Adak**

Patient **Shailesh Pethani from Mumbai** age **55 yrs reported** to N.I.C.E with the symptoms of **Fever, Sore throat** on 20-Jun-20 got cured in **7 days** under the N.I.C.E Care of **Sanjay Dhaduk**

Patient **Shubham Mishra** from **Delhi** age **24 yrs reported** to N.I.C.E with the symptoms of **Fever, Tiredness** on 23-Jun-20 got cured in **6 days** under the N.I.C.E Care of **Goma Ram**

Patient **Bal krishna** from **Mumbai** age **51 yrs reported** to N.I.C.E with the symptoms of **Dry Cough, Sore throat, Body ache/muscle ache, Tiredness, breathing difficulty** on **01-Jul-20** got cured in **3 days** under the N.I.C.E Care of **Kamal Dhawan**

Patient **Prince** from **Surat** age **32 yrs reported** to N.I.C.E with the symptoms of **Fever, Tiredness** on 02-Jul-20 got cured in **3 days** under the N.I.C.E Care of **Sushma Bengani**

Patient **Navin Singhi** from **Kolkata** age **29 yrs reported** to N.I.C.E with the symptoms of **Fever, Body ache/muscle ache, Tiredness** on **19-Jun-20** got cured in **7 days** under the N.I.C.E Care of **Chitra Jain**

Patient **Amit Singhi** from **Kolkata** age **29 yrs reported** to N.I.C.E with the symptoms of Fever, **Body ache/muscle ache, Tiredness** on **19-Jun-20** got cured in **6 days** under the N.I.C.E Care of **Sayed shah**

Patient **Sanjeev Kumar** from **Delhi** age **49 yrs reported** to N.I.C.E with the symptom of **Tiredness** on **11-Jun-20** got cured in **6 days** under the N.I.C.E Care of **Raushan Kumar**

Patient **Sohel Siddiqui** from **Mumbai** age **27 yrs reported** to N.I.C.E with the symptom of **Fever** on **12-Jun-20 got** cured in **4 days** under the N.I.C.E Care of **Madhuri Anad Kinikar**

Patient **Dheeraj Oberoi** from **New delhi** age **25 yrs reported** to N.I.C.E with the symptoms of **Fever, Headache, Body ache/muscle ache, Tiredness** on **13-Jun-20** got cured in **6 days** under the N.I.C.E Care of **Pratik Anand**

Patient **Shubham Khairnar** from **Aurangabad** age **24 yrs reported** to N.I.C.E with the symptom of **Congestion** on **30-Jun-20** got cured in **6 days** under the N.I.C.E Care of **Karan Shetty**

Patient **Swami Prasad Pal** from **Bhubaneswar** age **46 yrs reported** to N.I.C.E with the symptoms of **Dry Cough, Sore throat, Tirednes**son **27-Jun-20 got** cured in **5 days** under the N.I.C.E Care of **Sayed Shah**

Patient **Om Prakash** from **New Delhi** age **58 yrs reported** to N.I.C.E with the symptom of **Fever** on **10-Jun-20** got cured in **6 days** under the N.I.C.E Care of **Shaikh Warisha Nasim**

Patient **Hemant Bindal** from **New Delhi** age **28 yrs reported** to N.I.C.E with the symptoms of Fever, **Dry Cough, Sore throat, Headache, Body ache/muscle ache, Congestion, Tiredness, breathing difficulty** on **11-Jun-20** got cured in **7 days** under the N.I.C.E Care of **Emandi Kumar Rao**

Patient **Subrata chakrabarty** from **Bhubaneswar** age 41 **yrs reported** to N.I.C.E with the symptom of Dry **Cough** on 30-**Jun-20 got** cured in **7 days** under the N.I.C.E Care of **Mansi Thaker**

Patient **Sudhir Shinde** from **Mumbai** age 35 yrs reported to N.I.C.E with the symptoms of Fever, **Dry Cough, Sore throat, Headache, Body ache/muscle ache**on **02-Jul-20** got cured in **6 days** under the

N.I.C.E Care of **Shaikh Warisha Nasim**

Patient **Sunil Chatterjee** from **Ahmedabad** age 53 **yrs reported** to N.I.C.E with the symptoms of Fever, **Dry Cough, Headache, Body ache/muscle ache, breathing difficulty** on 23-Jun- 20 **got** cured in **6 days** under the N.I.C.E Care of **Lomash Anand**

Patient **Md Jameel** from **Hyderabad** age **50 yrs reported** to N.I.C.E with the symptoms of **Fever, Dry Cough, Body ache/muscle ache, Congestion, Tiredness, breathing difficulty** on 16-Jun-20 **got** cured in **5 days** under the N.I.C.E Care of **Kamal Dhawan**

Patient **Sumit Sharma** from **Meerut** age **26 yrs reported** to N.I.C.E with the symptoms of **Fever, Headache** on 17-Jun-20 **got** cured in **3 days** under the N.I.C.E Care of **Shreya Gadiya**

Patient **Anju Gupta** from **Faridabad** age 54 **yrs reported** to N.I.C.E with the symptoms of **Dry Cough, Sore throat, Headache, Body ache/muscle ache, Congestion, Tiredness, breathing difficulty** on 03-Jul-20 **got** cured in **7 days** under the N.I.C.E Care of **Dr. Barin Kumar Roy**

Patient **Sunil Kuma** rfrom **Ghaziabad** age **30 yrs reported** to N.I.C.E with the symptoms of **Headache, breathing difficulty** on 26-Jun-20 **got** cured in **4 days** under the N.I.C.E Care of **Raushan Kumar**

Patient **Himanshu Pathak**from **Ghaziabad** age **33 yrs reported** to N.I.C.E with the symptoms of **Fever, Sore throat, Headache, Body ache/muscle ache** on 24-Jun-20 **got** cured in **7 days** under the N.I.C.E Care of **Ritu Singh**

Patient **Sunny** from **Sonipat** age **34 yrs reported** to N.I.C.E with the symptom of Sore **throat** on 25-Jun-20 got cured in **4 days** under the N.I.C.E Care of **BrijmohanYadav**

Patient **Siddhant B Upadeshe** from **Kalyan** age 28 **yrs reported** to N.I.C.E with the symptoms of Fever, **Headache, and Body ache/ muscle ache** on 26-Jun-20 got cured in **3 days** under the N.I.C.E Care of **Suresh Kumar Yadav**

Patient **Surekha Jagtap** from **Mumbai** age 38 yrs **reported** to N.I.C.E with the symptoms of **Dry Cough, Headache, and Tiredness** on 26-Jun-20 got cured in **7 days** under the N.I.C.E Care of **Nishan Singh Jamwal**

Patient **Shushant Singh** from **Kanpur** age 33 yrs **reported** to N.I.C.E with the symptoms of **Body ache/muscle ache, Tiredness** on 29-Jun-20 got cured in **7 days** under the N.I.C.E Care of **Satish Kumar Varma Vuppalapati**

Patient **Sushil Kumar Doddi** from **Bhiwandi** age **38 yrs reported** to N.I.C.E with the symptoms of Headache, **Body ache/muscle ache, Tiredness** on 27-Jun-20 got cured in **5 days** under the N.I.C.E Care of **Gopinath Narayanam**

Patient **Suyog Saokhe** from **New Delhi** age **32 yrs reported** to N.I.C.E with the symptom of **breathing difficulty** on 11-Jun-20 got cured in **6 days** under the N.I.C.E Care of **Raushan Kumar**

Patient **Amit jain** from **Ranchi** age **39 yrs reported** to N.I.C.E with the symptom of **breathing difficulty on** 02-Jul- **20** got cured in 7 **days** under the N.I.C.E Care of **Samir Das**

Patient Prem **Grover** from **Mumbai** age **73yrs reported** to N.I.C.E with the symptoms of **Fever, Tiredness** on 18-Jun-20 got cured in **3 days** under the N.I.C.E Care of **Dr Seema Arora**

Patient **Syed Aziz** from **Hyderabad** age **45 yrs reported** to N.I.C.E with the symptoms of **Fever, Dry Cough, and breathing difficulty on** 17-Jun-20 got cured in **4 days** under the N.I.C.E Care of **Siddharth Jain**

Patient **Meena Handa from Delhi** age **58 yrs reported** to N.I.C.E with the symptoms of Fever, **Dry Cough, Sore throat, Headache, Body ache/muscle ache, Tiredness**on 12-Jun-20 **got** cured in 7 **days** under the N.I.C.E Care of **Hemraj Jagannath Saner**

Patient **Virendra** from **Gurugram** age **49yrs**yrs reported to N.I.C.E with the symptoms of **Fever, Headache, Body ache/muscle ache,**

Tiredness on 09-**Jun-20 got** cured in **6 days** under the N.I.C.E Care of **Kunwar Aryaman**

Patient **Dr. Deepak Tomar** from **Gurugram** age **39 yrs reported** to N.I.C.E with the symptoms of **Fever, Body ache/muscle ache** on 17-**Jun-20 got** cured in **7 days** under the N.I.C.E Care of **Dr. Atul Ramesh Arkhede**

Patient **Gopal Krishnan** from **Mumbai** age **68 yrs reported** to N.I.C.E with the symptoms of **Fever, Headache, Body ache/muscle ache, Tiredness** on **02-Jul-20** got cured in **3 days** under the N.I.C.E Care of **Ajeet Singh**

Patient **Shweta Jain** from **Rohini** age **26 yrs reported** to N.I.C.E with the symptom of **Fever** on 23-**Jun-20 got** cured in **7 days** under the N.I.C.E Care of **Dr. Kishan Pareek**

Patient **Sakshi Jain** from **Bhind** age **21 yrs reported** to N.I.C.E with the symptoms of **Fever, Dry Cough, Headache, Body ache/ muscle ache, Tiredness** on 23-**Jun-20 got** cured in **7 days** under the N.I.C.E Care of **Dr. Lakshmi Narayan Reddy**

Patient **Sourabh Jain** from **Bhind** age **29 yrs reported** to N.I.C.E with the symptoms of **Fever, Sore throat, Tiredness** on 14-**Jun-20 got** cured in **3 days** under the N.I.C.E Care of **Simi Handa**

Patient **Dr Varun** from **New Delhi** age **40 yrs reported** to N.I.C.E with the symptoms of **Body ache/muscle ache, Tiredness** on 11-**Jun-20** got cured in **6 days** under the N.I.C.E Care of **Jitendra Kumar Choubey**

Patient **Arti Sharma** from **Delhi** age **31 yrs reported** to N.I.C.E with the symptoms of **Headache, Body ache/muscle ache, Tiredness** on 08-**Jun-20 got** cured in **3 days** under the N.I.C.E Care of **Shikha Saxena**

Patient **Jai** from **Delhi** age **2 yrs reported** to N.I.C.E with the symptom of **Fever, Dry Cough** on 12-**Jun-20 got** cured in **6 days** under the N.I.C.E Care of **Daniyal Mujawar**

Patient **Sanju Kumari** from **Noida** age **27** yrs reported to N.I.C.E with the symptom of **Fever** on **29-Jun-20** got cured in **7 days** under the N.I.C.E Care of **Ritu Singh**

Patient **Vijay** from **Mumbai** age **50 yrs reported** to N.I.C.E with the symptom of **Sore throat** on 25-**Jun-20** got cured in **4 days** under the N.I.C.E Care of **Shreya Gadiya**

Patient Rakhi **Ravindra Sawant** from **Mumbai borivali** age **33 yrs reported** to N.I.C.E with the symptoms of Dry **Cough, Headache, Body ache/muscle ache, Congestion, Tiredness** on 25-Jun-20 got cured in **7 days** under the N.I.C.E Care of **Arun Kumar**

Patient **Vijoy K Prasad** from **Shyam Nagar** age **33 yrs reported** to N.I.C.E with the symptom of **Fever** on 25-**Jun-20** got cured in **5 days** under the N.I.C.E Care of **Bimal Pal**

Patient **Vinod Kumar** from **New Delhi** age **49 yrs reported** to N.I.C.E with the symptom of **Sore throat** on 24-**Jun-20** got cured in **5 days** under the N.I.C.E Care of **Dr. C Rajasekhar**

Patient **Vandna Doutani** from **Delhi** age **42 yrs reported** to N.I.C.E with the symptom of **breathing difficulty** on 29-**Jun-20** got cured in **7 days** under the N.I.C.E Care of **Bhagwan Dass**

Patient **Vinod Kumar** from **New Delhi** age 31 **yrs reported** to N.I.C.E with the symptoms of Dry **Cough, Sore throat, Tiredness, breathing difficulty** on 27-**Jun-20 got** cured in **5 days** under the N.I.C.E Care of **Renu Garg**

Patient **Megha Jain** from **Delhi** age 40 **yrs reported** to N.I.C.E with the symptoms of Fever, **Sore throat, Headache, Body ache/muscle ache, Tiredness, breathing difficulty** on 15-Jun-20 got cured in **6 days** under the N.I.C.E Care of **Arvind Kumar Plaha**

Patient **Shelly Jain** from **Delhi** age 1 **yrs reported** to N.I.C.E with the symptoms of Fever, **Sore throat, Headache, Body ache/muscle ache, Tiredness** on 24-**Jun-20 got** cured in **3 days** under the N.I.C.E Care of **Milesh Sahare**

Patient **Sukh Dev Soni** from **Faridabad** age **64 yrs reported** to N.I.C.E with the symptoms of **Fever, Dry Cough, and Sore throat** on 19-**Jun-20** got cured in **4 days** under the N.I.C.E Care of **Kanishk Amarpuri**

Patient **Sushma Verma** from **New Delhi** age **49 yrs reported** to N.I.C.E with the symptoms of **Dry Cough, Congestion, breathing difficulty on** 24-**Jun-20 got** cured in **3 days** under the N.I.C.E Care of **Ritu Singh**

Patient **Ritika Ahuja** from **Faridabad** age **31 yrs reported** to N.I.C.E with the symptoms of **Fever, Dry Cough, Headache, Tiredness** on 13-**Jun-20** got cured in **5 days** under the N.I.C.E Care of **Rupesh Umar**

Patient **kawleen** from **New delhi** age 31 **yrs reported** to N.I.C.E with the symptoms of Sore **throat, Body ache/muscle ache, Tiredness** on 25-**Jun-20 got** cured in **3 days** under the N.I.C.E Care of **Sounak Das**

Patient **Lalit Kumar** from **Ghaziabad** age 44 **yrs reported** to N.I.C.E with the symptoms of Fever**, Dry Cough, and Sore throat** on 25-**Jun-20 got** cured in **6 days** under the N.I.C.E Care of **Baltej Singh**

Patient **Sanjay Sharma from Mathabhanga** age 57 **yrs reported** to N.I.C.E with the symptoms of Fever, **Body ache/muscle ache, Tiredness** on 24-**Jun-20** got cured in **3 days** under the N.I.C.E Care of **Ashok N Adak**

Patient **Akshata Yashwant Shinde** from **Mumbai** age 23 **yrs reported** to N.I.C.E with the symptom of Fever on 29-**Jun-20** got cured in **4 days** under the N.I.C.E Care of **Sounak Das**

Patient **Yashwant B Wakkar** from **Mumbai** age 50 yrs **reported** to N.I.C.E with the symptoms of Fever**, Dry Cough, Body ache/ muscle ache, Tiredness** on 28-**Jun-20** got cured in **7 days** under the N.I.C.E Care of **Ritu Singh**

Patient **Yasin Shaikh** from **Nashik** age 24yrs **reported** to N.I.C.E with the symptoms of Fever**, Headache, Body ache/muscle ache, Congestion, Tiredness** on 26-**Jun-20 got** cured in **3 days** under the N.I.C.E Care of **Kunwar Aryaman**

Patient **Yogesh Kumar** from **Delhi** age 43 **yrs reported** to N.I.C.E with the symptoms of Fever**, Sore throat** on 13-**Jun-20** got cured in **7 days** under the N.I.C.E Care of **Mushtaque Ahmad**

Patient **Mushtari Begum** from **Kolkata** age 60 yrs **reported** to N.I.C.E with the symptoms of Fever**, Dry Cough, Headache, Body ache/muscle ache, Tiredness** on 27-**Jun-20** got cured in **4 days** under the N.I.C.E Care of **Ajit Kumar Burnwal**

Patient **Kirti Posture** from **Mumbai** age 31 **yrs reported** to N.I.C.E with the symptoms of Fever**, Body ache/muscle ache, Tiredness** on 18-**Jun-20** got cured in **days** under the N.I.C.E Care of **Bhagwan Das**

Patient **Ashok R. Nikalje** from **Pune** age 54 **yrs reported** to N.I.C.E with the symptoms of Fever**, Body ache/muscle ache, Tiredness** on 24-**Jun-20** got cured in **days** under the N.I.C.E Care of **Pradeep Chauhan**

Patient **Sonal Ben Sodvadiya** from **Surat** age 34 **yrs reported** to N.I.C.E with the symptoms of Fever**, Sore throat, Headache, Body ache/muscle ache** on 24-**Jun-20** got cured in **days** under the N.I.C.E Care of **Ashok N Adak**

Patient **Shivam Vishwakarma** from **Delhi** age 21 **yrs reported** to N.I.C.E with the symptoms of Fever**, Headache, Body ache/muscle ache, Tiredness** on 30-**Jun-20** got cured in **days** under the N.I.C.E Care of **Ashok N Adak**

Patient **Suhas Gopal Thorat** from **Panvel** age 40 **yrs reported** to N.I.C.E with the symptoms of Fever**, Dry Cough, and Sore throat** on 30-**Jun-20** got cured in **days** under the N.I.C.E Care of **Ashok N Adak**

Patient **Sanjay Sharma** from **Nashik** age 57 yrs **reported** to N.I.C.E with the symptoms of Fever, **Body ache/muscle ache, Tiredness** on 24-**Jun-20** got cured in **days** under the N.I.C.E Care of **Ashok N Adak**

Patient **Shashiraj** from **Kurukshetra** age **36 yrs reported** to N.I.C.E with the symptoms of Fever, **Sore throat, Tiredness** on 24-Jun-20 got cured in **days** under the N.I.C.E Care of **Ashok N Adak**

Patient **Manoj Mishra** from **Delhi** age 32yrs **reported** to N.I.C.E with the symptoms of Fever, **Headache, and breathing difficulty** on 16-**Jun-20** got cured in **days** under the N.I.C.E Care of **Lomash anand**

Patient **Jagdish Sharma** from **Bhiwani** age 33 **yrs reported** to N.I.C.E with the symptoms of Fever, **Dry Cough, Body ache/ muscle ache** on 16-**Jun-20** got cured in **days** under the N.I.C.E Care of **Lomash Anand**

Patient **Anju Gupta** from **Faridabad** age **54yrs reported** to N.I.C.E with the symptoms of **Dry Cough, Sore throat, Headache, Body ache/muscle ache, Congestion, Tiredness, Breathing difficulty** on **03-Jul-20** got cured in **days** under the N.I.C.E Care of **Dr. Barin Kumar Roy**

Patient **Fareeha** from **Hyderabad** age 14 **yrs reported** to N.I.C.E with the symptom of Dry **Cough** on 03-**Jul-20** got cured in **days** under the N.I.C.E Care of **Dr. Barin Kumar Roy**

Patient **Shaluta Sandeep Lahane** from **Thane** age 36 **yrs reported** to N.I.C.E with the symptom of Fever on 22-**Jun-20** got cured in **days** under the N.I.C.E Care of **Dr. Barin Kumar Roy**

Patient **Manish Saluja** from **Surat** age 35 **yrs reported** to N.I.C.E with the symptoms of **Fever, Sore throat, Headache, Body ache/ muscle ache, Tiredness** on 21-**Jun-20 got** cured in **days** under the N.I.C.E Care of **Gopinath Narayanam**

Patient **Gaurav Goel** from **Noida** age 48 **yrs reported** to N.I.C.E with the symptoms of Fever, **Dry Cough, and Sore throat** on 03-

Jul-20 got cured in **days** under the N.I.C.E Care of **Nishu Sandhya**

Patient **Narendra Jadav** from **Ahmedabad** age **27 yrs reported** to N.I.C.E with the symptoms of **Headache, Breathing difficulty** on **25-Jun-20** got cured in **days** under the N.I.C.E Care of **Satish Kumar Varma Vuppalapati**

Patient **Atul Jain** from **Delhi** age **48 yrs reported** to N.I.C.E with the symptoms of **Dry Cough, Headache, Tiredness** on **25-Jun-20** got cured in **days** under the N.I.C.E Care of **Satish Kumar Varma Vuppalapati**

Patient **Sandeep Dhabolkar** from **Mumbai** age **40 yrs reported** to N.I.C.E with the symptoms of Fever, **Sore throat, Body ache/ muscle ache, Tiredness** on 24-**Jun-20 got** cured in **days** under the N.I.C.E Care of **Narendra Singh Patel**

Patient **Basilal Ramesh** from **Hyderabad** age **67yrs reported** to N.I.C.E with the symptoms of Fever, **Dry Cough, breathing difficulty** on **04-Jul-20** got cured in **days** under the N.I.C.E Care of **Dr Pankaj Chaudhary**

Patient **Vandna Jain** from **Delhi** age **42 yrs reported** to N.I.C.E with the symptoms of Fever, **Body ache/muscle ache** on **17-Jun-20** got cured in **days** under the N.I.C.E Care of **Prabhjot Kaur**

Patient **Dinesh Kumar** from **New Delhi** age **47 yrs reported** to N.I.C.E with the symptoms of Fever, **Dry Cough, Body ache/ muscle ache, Congestion** on 17-**Jun-20** got cured in **days** under the N.I.C.E Care of **Prabhjot Kaur**

Patient **Navin Goel** from **New Delhi** age 64 yrs reported to N.I.C.E with the suspected symptoms of Influenza/**flu** on **17-Jun-20** with co- morbidity like **Diabetes** got cured in **4 days** under the N.I.C.E Care of **Chitra Jain.**

Patient **Arvind** from **Ulhasnagar** age 40 **yrs reported** to N.I.C.E with the suspected symptoms of Influenza/**flu** on **20-Jun-20**with co -morbidity like **Thyroid** got cured in **4** days under the N.I.C.E Care of **Biswajit Datta.**

Patient **Pramod** from **Mumbai** age 63 yrs reported to N.I.C.E with the suspected symptoms of Influenza/**flu** on **21-Jun-20** with co-morbidity like **Achilles Tendonitis** got cured in **6** days under the N.I.C.E Care of **Sunita Dolley.**

Patient **Priya Pawaskar** from Thane age 31 **yrs reported** to N.I.C.E with the suspected symptoms of Influenza/**flu** on **20-Jun-20** with co- morbidities like **High BP & hypothyroid** got cured in **3** days under the N.I.C.E Care of **Dharmendra Kumar Pandey.**

Patient **Satyeshva** from **Navi Mumbai** age 53 **yrs reported** to N.I.C.E with the suspected symptoms of Influenza/**flu** on **18-Jun-20** with co- morbidity like **BP** got cured in **3** days under the N.I.C.E Care of **Dr. Kishan Pareek.**

Patient **Rajendra** from **Kaman** age 32 **yrs reported** to N.I.C.E with the suspected symptoms of Influenza/**flu** on **18-Jun-20** with co-morbidity like Sinus got cured in **4** days under the N.I.C.E Care of **Shiv Dular.**

Patient **Shrihaan Vashista** from **New Delhi** age 3months yrs reported to N.I.C.E with the suspected symptoms of Influenza/**flu** on **30-Jun-20** got cured in **4** days the N.I.C.E Care of **Kamlakshi Shahdeo**

Patient **Sameer Vilas Verulkar** from **Mumbai** age 32 yrs reported to N.I.C.E with the suspected symptoms of Influenza/**flu** on **08-Jul-20** got cured in **3** days the N.I.C.E Care of **Savio Paes**

Patient S**angeeta Chopra** from **Gurugram** age 39 yrs reported to N.I.C.E with the suspected symptoms of Influenza/**flu** on **03-Jul-20** got cured in **5** days the N.I.C.E Care of Nishu **Sandhya**

Patient **Shivanath Gupta** from **Bilaspur** age 1 yr **reported** to N.I.C.E with the symptoms of Fever, **Dry Cough, and Tiredness** on 19-**Jun- 20** got cured in **6 days** under the N.I.C.E Care of **Sudhir Kumar**

Patient **Gaurav Maruti Jadhav** from **Mumbai** age 29 **yrs reported** to N.I.C.E with the symptoms of Fever, **Dry Cough, Headache,**

Body ache/muscle ache, Congestion, Tiredness, breathing difficulty on 22-Jun-20 got cured in **6 days** under the N.I.C.E Care of **Dr. Vishwajeet Khaiwal**

Patient **Rajesh Luthra** from **Delhi** age 46 **yrs reported** to N.I.C.E with the symptoms of Fever, **Sore throat, Body ache/muscle ache, Congestion, Tiredness** on 26-Jun-20 got cured in **4 days** under the N.I.C.E Care of **Filda Don**

Patient **Sudhir** from **Delhi** age 61 **yrs reported** to N.I.C.E with the symptoms of Fever, **Tiredness** on 13-Jun-20 got cured in **7 days** under the N.I.C.E Care of **Bhagwan Dass**

Patient **Rajanikant Eknath Chavan** from **Kalyan** age 26 **yrs reported** to N.I.C.E with the symptoms of Body **ache/muscle ache** on 27-**Jun-20** got cured in **4 days** under the N.I.C.E Care of **Ashish**

Patient **Manish Thorat** from **Mumbai** age 33 **yrs reported** to N.I.C.E with the symptom of **breathing difficulty** on 27-**Jun-20 got** cured in **3 days** under the N.I.C.E Care of **Arvind Kumar Plaha**

Patient **Iqbal Singh** from **New Delhi** age 28yrs **reported** to N.I.C.E with the symptoms of Fever, **Body ache/muscle ache, Tiredness** on 17-**Jun-20** got cured in **6 days** under the N.I.C.E Care of **Prabin Nanda**

Patient **Ramchandra Dongale** from **Dombivali** age 34yrs **reported** to N.I.C.E with the symptoms of **Fever, Body ache/muscle ache** on 02-**Jul-20** got cured in **3 days** under the N.I.C.E Care of **Dr Seema Arora**

Patient **Rama Sharma** from **Delhi** age 34yrs **reported** to N.I.C.E with the symptoms of Fever, **Dry Cough, Sore throat, Body ache/ muscle ache, Tiredness, breathing difficulty** on 21-Jun-20 got cured in **7 days** under the N.I.C.E Care of **Chitra Jain**

Patient **Rashmi Ranjan Jena** from **New Delhi** age 36 **yrs reported** to N.I.C.E with the symptoms of Dry **Cough, Sore throat, Tiredness** on 29-Jun-20 got cured in **4 days** under the N.I.C.E Care of **Bhagwan Dass**

Patient **Kalavati Budharapu** from **Mumbai** age 54 **yrs reported** to N.I.C.E with the symptoms of **breathing difficulty** on 10-**Jun-20** got cured in **5 days** under the N.I.C.E Care of **Prabin Nanda**

Patient **Reena** from **Siwani** age **28 yrs reported** to N.I.C.E with the symptoms of Fever**, Headache, Body ache/muscle ache, Tiredness** on 11-**Jun-20** got cured in **6 days** under the N.I.C.E Care of **Sayed Shah**

Patient **Ms Rehnuma** from **New Delhi** age 32 **yrs reported** to N.I.C.E with the symptoms of **Congestion, loss of taste or smell** on 06-**Jun-20** got cured in **5 days** under the N.I.C.E Care of **Gaurav Jain**

Patient **Durgesh Gupta** from **Gurugram** age 38yrs **reported** to N.I.C.E with the symptoms of Fever**, Dry Cough, Sore throat, Headache, Body ache/muscle ache, breathing difficulty** on 20-**Jun-20** got cured in **4 days** under the N.I.C.E Care of **Dr. Kishan Pareek**

Patient **Rahul Gupta** from **Gurugram** age **30 yrs reported** to N.I.C.E with the symptoms of Fever**, Dry Cough, Body ache/ muscle ache** on 20-**Jun-20** got cured in **7 days** under the N.I.C.E Care of **Kamal Dhawan**

Patient **Rinku Barua** from **Faridabad** age 44 **yrs reported** to N.I.C.E with the symptoms of Fever on 26-**Jun-20** got cured in **4 days** under the N.I.C.E Care of Gopinath **Narayanam**

Patient **Manish Sharma** from **Bengaluru** age 41 **yrs reported** to N.I.C.E with the symptoms of Sore **Throat, Jaw pain salivary gland infection** on 06-**Jun-20** got cured in **7 days** under the N.I.C.E Care of **Kapil Dev Sharma**

Patient **Arti** from **Bhopal** age 45 **yrs reported** to N.I.C.E with the symptoms of Fever**, Sore throat, Body ache/muscle ache, Tiredness** on 16-**Jun-20** got cured in **7 days** under the N.I.C.E Care of **Dr. Kishan Pareek**

Patient **Ruchi** from **Delhi** age 38 **yrs reported** to N.I.C.E with the symptoms of Fever, **Sore throat** on 20-**Jun-20** got cured in **7 days** under the N.I.C.E Care of **Ajit Kumar Burnwal**

Patient **Mohini Gautom** from **Delhi age** 29 **yrs reported** to N.I.C.E with the symptoms of Fever, **Dry Cough, Headache, Body ache/ muscle ache, Tiredness** on 25-Jun-20 got cured in **6 days** under the N.I.C.E Care of **Dr.Narasinha Swami Mamdyal**

Patient **Yadav Hrishikesh** from **Thane** age 20 **yrs reported** to N.I.C.E with the symptoms of **Fever, breathing difficulty** on 27-Jun-20 got cured in **7 days** under the N.I.C.E Care of **Jasmeet Kaur**

Patient **Shraddha** from **Mumbai** age 27 **yrs reported** to N.I.C.E with the symptoms of Fever, **Sore throat** on 26-Jun-20 got cured in **3 days** under the N.I.C.E Care of **Dr Rajendra Prasad Kumawat**

Patient **Sagar Rane** from **Mumbai** age 37 **yrs reported** to N.I.C.E with the symptom of Body **ache/muscle ache** on 18-Jun-20 got cured in **5 days** under the N.I.C.E Care of **Samir Das**

Patient **Saggu Sarabjit Kaur** from **Ghaziabad** age 44 **yrs reported** to N.I.C.E with the symptoms of **Fever, Dry Cough, Sore throat, Body ache/muscle ache, Tiredness** on 17-Jun-20 got cured in **5 days** under the N.I.C.E Care of **Siddharth Jain**

Patient **Sajal Nandagawli** from **Pune** age 27 **yrs reported** to N.I.C.E with the symptoms of Dry **Cough, Sore throat, Body ache/muscle ache, Congestion, Tiredness, breathing difficulty** on 27-Jun-20 got cured in **3 days** under the N.I.C.E Care of **Arvind Kumar Plaha**

Patient **Aleem Ansari** from **Telengana** age 56 **yrs** reported to N.I.C.E with the symptoms of Fever, **Dry Cough, and breathing difficulty** on 29-Jun-20 got cured in **3 days** under the N.I.C.E Care of **Sounak Das**

Patient **Salim Vohra** from **Mumbai** age 64 **yrs reported** to N.I.C.E with the symptom of Body **ache/muscle ache** on 01-Jul-20 got cured in **6 days** under the N.I.C.E Care of **Rajeev Kumar**

Patient **Nishid Prithviraj** from Thane age 24 **yrs reported** to N.I.C.E with the symptoms of Fever, **Dry Cough, Sore throat, Headache, Body ache/muscle ache** on **01-Jul-20** got cured in **3 days** under the N.I.C.E Care of **Alisha Massey**

Patient **Sameer Shaikh** from **Pune** age 44 **yrs reported** to N.I.C.E with the symptoms of Fever, **Body ache/muscle ache** on **21-Jun-20** got cured in **3 days** under the N.I.C.E Care of **Kamal Dhawan**

Patient **Sulekha** from **Delhi** age 48 **yrs reported** to N.I.C.E with the symptoms of Fever, **Headache, and Tiredness** on **26-Jun-20 got** cured in **7 days** under the N.I.C.E Care of **Jitendra Kumar Choubey**

Patient **Sameer Vilas Verulkar** from **Mumbai** age 37 **yrs reported** to N.I.C.E with **suspected symptoms of influenza** on **08-Jul-20** got cured in **6 days** under the N.I.C.E Care of **Savio Paes**

Patient **Safurah Anam** from **Hyderabad** age 14 yrs reported to N.I.C.E with the symptoms of Sore **throat, Body ache/muscle ache, Tiredness, breathing difficulty** on **29-Jun-20** got cured in **7 days** under the N.I.C.E Care of **Milesh Sahare**

Patient **Samrat Sethia** from **Mumbai** age 44 **yrs reported** to N.I.C.E with the symptoms of Fever, **Sore throat, Headache, Body ache/ muscle ache** on **13-Jun-20** got cured in **6 days** under the N.I.C.E Care of **Kapil Dev Sharma**

Patient **Aradhika Chopra** from **Allahabad** age 60 **yrs reported** to N.I.C.E with the symptoms of Fever, **Tiredness** on **18-Jun-20** got cured in **6 days** under the N.I.C.E Care of **Dr Seema Arora**

Patient **Sharwan Kumar** from **Biharsharif** age 55 **yrs reported** to N.I.C.E with the symptoms of Fever, **Body ache/muscle ache, Tiredness** on **01-Jul-20** got cured in **5 days** under the N.I.C.E Care of **Dr. Barin Kumar Roy**

Patient **Sandeep Goyal** from **Ghaziabad** age 47 **yrs reported** to N.I.C.E with the symptoms of Fever, **Headache, Body ache/muscle** ache, **Tiredness** on 29-**Jun-20** got cured in **6 days** under the N.I.C.E Care of **Dr Seema Arora**

Patient **Sandeep Garg** from **Vikas puri** age 44 **yrs reported** to N.I.C.E with the symptom of Fever on 30-**Jun-20** got cured in **3 days** under the N.I.C.E Care of **Samir Das**

Patient **Sanjesh Ahuja** from **Noida** age 57 **yrs reported** to N.I.C.E with the symptoms of Sore **throat, Tiredness** on 11-**Jun-20** got cured in **7 days** under the N.I.C.E Care of **Punyaapriya**

Patient **Santhosh Tomar** from **Mandideep** age 44 **yrs reported** to N.I.C.E with the symptoms of Fever, **Body ache/muscle ache** on 27-**Jun-20** got cured in **6 days** under the N.I.C.E Care of **Mansi Thaker**

Patient **Santosh Kumar Sinha** from **South Delhi** age 36 **yrs reported** to N.I.C.E with the symptoms of Fever, **Sore throat** on 26-**Jun-20** got cured in **6 days** under the N.I.C.E Care of **Biswajit Datta**

Patient **Sarika Arora** from **New Delhi** age 38 **yrs reported** to N.I.C.E with the symptoms of Fever, **Dry Cough, Sore throat, Body ache/ muscle ache, breathing difficulty** on 19-**Jun-20** got cured in **7 days** under the N.I.C.E Care of **Ananta Kumar Panda**

Patient **Vibhuti Yadav** from **Delhi** age 20 **yrs reported** to N.I.C.E with the symptoms of Fever on 12-**Jun-20** got cured in **7 days** under the N.I.C.E Care of **Sounak Das**

Patient **Satinder Singh** from **Secunderabad** age 36 **yrs reported** to N.I.C.E with the symptoms of Fever, **Body ache/muscle ache** on 28-**Jun-20** got cured in **3 days** under the N.I.C.E Care of **Kanishk Amarpuri**

Patient **Manish saluja** from **Surat** age 35 **yrs** reported to N.I.C.E with the symptoms of **Fever, Sore throat, Headache, Body ache/ muscle ache, Tiredness** on 21-**Jun-20** got cured in **7 days** under the N.I.C.E Care of **Gopinath Narayanam**

Patient **Irshad** from **Anantapur** age **46 yrs** reported to N.I.C.E with the symptoms of **Fever, Dry Cough, Headache** on **02-Jul-20** got cured in **6 days** under the N.I.C.E Care of **Nilima N Bhatkar**

Patient **Ankesh** from **Greater Noida** age **27 yrs** reported to N.I.C.E with the symptoms of **Fever, Headache, Breathing difficulty** on **29-Jun-20** got cured in **5 days** under the N.I.C.E Care of **Nilima N Bhatkar**

Patient **Urbashi Shaw** from **Dehradun** age **31 yrs** reported to N.I.C.E with the symptoms of **Nasal irritation** on **06-Jul-20** got cured in **6 days** under the N.I.C.E Care of **Sounak Das**

Patient **Umesh Sharma** from **Panvel** age **46 yrs** reported to N.I.C.E with the symptoms of **Fever, Dry Cough** on **24-Jun-20** got cured in **4 days** under the N.I.C.E Care of **Narendra Singh Patel**

Patient **Vidya Bharat Kumar ambati** from **Nerul** age **31 yrs** reported to N.I.C.E with the symptoms of **Sore throat** on **06-Jul-20** got cured in **6 days** under the N.I.C.E Care of **Gopinath Narayanam**

Patient **Simi Handa** from **New Delhi** age **28 yrs** reported to N.I.C.E with the symptoms of **Fever, Dry Cough, Body ache/muscle ache, Tiredness,** on **21-Jun-20** got cured in **4 days** under the N.I.C.E Care of **Simi Handa**

Patient **Gaurav Goyal** from **Noida** age **48 yrs** reported to N.I.C.E with the symptoms of **Fever, Dry Cough, Sore throat** on **03-Jul-20** got cured in **6 days** under the N.I.C.E Care of **Nishu Sandhya**

Patient **Mohammad Iqbal** from **Muharraq - Bahrain** age **42 yrs** reported to N.I.C.E with the symptoms of **Fever, Tiredness** on **07-Feb-20** got cured in **5 days** under the N.I.C.E Care of **Rajwinder Kaur**

Patient **Narendra Jadav** from **Ahmedabad** age **27 yrs** reported to N.I.C.E with the symptoms of **Headache, breathing difficulty** on **25-Jun-20** got cured in **7 days** under the N.I.C.E Care of **Satish Kumar Varma Vuppalapati**

Patient **Atul Jain** from **New Delhi** age **48 yrs** reported to N.I.C.E with the symptoms of **Dry Cough, Headache, Tiredness** on **25-Jun-20** got cured in **7 days** under the N.I.C.E Care of **Satish Kumar Varma Vuppalapati**

Patient **Sandeep Dhabolkar** from **Mumbai** age **40 yrs** reported to N.I.C.E with the symptoms of **Fever, Sore throat, Body ache/ muscle ache, Tiredness** on **24-Jun-20** got cured in **6 days** under the N.I.C.E Care of **Narendra Singh Patel**

Patient **Basilal Ramesh** from **Hyderabad** age **67 yrs** reported to N.I.C.E with the symptoms of **Fever,Dry Cough, Breathing difficulty** on **04-Jul-20** got cured in **4 days** under the N.I.C.E Care of **Dr Pankaj Chaudhary**

Patient **Vandna Jain** from **New Delhi** age **42 yrs** reported to N.I.C.E with the symptoms of **Fever, Body ache/muscle ache** on **17-Jun-20** got cured in **7 days** under the N.I.C.E Care of **Prabhjot Kaur**

Patient **Dinesh Kumar** from **New Delhi** age **47 yrs** reported to N.I.C.E with the symptoms of **Fever, Dry Cough, Body ache/ muscle ache, Congestion** on **17-Jun-20** got cured in **5 days** under the N.I.C.E Care of **Prabhjot Kaur**

Patient **Lewis Fernandes** from **Kuwait** age **12 yrs** reported to N.I.C.E with the symptoms of **Dry Cough, Sore throat, Body ache/ muscle ache,Congestion/, Tiredness, Weakness** on **07-Jul-20** got cured in **7 days** under the N.I.C.E Care of **Savio Paes**

Patient **Dinesh Kumar** from **Thane** age **35 yrs** reported to N.I.C.E with the symptoms of **Dry Cough, Body ache/muscle ache, Tiredness** on **20-Jun-20** got cured in **4 days** under the N.I.C.E Care of **Prabhjot Kaur**

Patient **Hitesh Lapsiwala** from **Surat** age **49 yrs** reported to N.I.C.E with the symptoms of **Fever, Headache, Body ache/muscle ache, Tiredness** on **03-Jul-20** got cured in **7 days** under the N.I.C.E Care of **Prabhjot Kaur**

Patient **Manish Nirwan** from **New Delhi** age **39 yrs** reported to N.I.C.E with the symptoms of **Fever, breathing difficulty** on 21-**Jun-20** got cured in **4 days** under the N.I.C.E Care of **Prabhjot Kaur**

Patient **Chandan** from **Pune** age **41 yrs** reported to N.I.C.E with the symptoms of **Dry Cough, Tiredness** on **01-Jul-20** got cured in **6 days** under the N.I.C.E Care of **Alisha Massey**

Patient **Yash singh** from **New Delhi** age **30 yrs** reported to N.I.C.E with the symptoms of **Fever, Sore throat, Body ache/muscle ache, Weakness** on **04-Jul-20** got cured in **3 days** under the N.I.C.E Care of **Nishu Sandhya**

Patient **Abhi** from **Pune** age **37 yrs** reported to N.I.C.E with the symptoms of **Fever, Weakness** on **07-Jun-20** got cured in **4 days** under the N.I.C.E Care of **Nishu Sandhya**

Patient **Munil Kumar** from **New Delhi** age **20 yrs** reported to N.I.C.E with the symptoms of **Fever, Headache, Tiredness** on **10-Jun-20** got cured in **3 days** under the N.I.C.E Care of **Shaikh Warisha Nasim**

Patient **Dharmender Kumar** from **New Delhi** age **46 yrs** reported to N.I.C.E with the symptoms of **Fever, Body ache/muscle ache, Tiredness** on **16-Jun-20** got cured in **3 days** under the N.I.C.E Care of **Hemraj Jagannath Saner**

Patient **Harman Singh** from **New Delhi** age **28 yrs** reported to N.I.C.E with the symptoms of **Fever, Dry Cough, Tiredness, Sore Throat, loss of taste or smell, Muscle and body aches** on **06-Jul-20** got cured in **1 day** under the N.I.C.E Care of **Ritu Singh**

Patient **Indu** from **New Delhi** age **31 yrs** reported to N.I.C.E with the symptoms of **Dry Cough, Headache, breathing difficulty** on **18-Jun-20** got cured in **7 days** under the N.I.C.E Care of **Brijmohan Yadav**

Patient **Anshul Garg** from **Hyderabad** age **26 yrs** reported to N.I.C.E with the symptoms of **Fever, Headache, breathing difficulty** on 21-

jun-20 got cured in **3 days** under the N.I.C.E Care of **Sounak Das**

Patient **Santosh Pandey** from **Ghaziabad** age **50 yrs** reported to N.I.C.E with the symptoms of **Fever, Headache, Body ache/muscle ache, Tiredness** got cured in **4 days** under the N.I.C.E Care of **Raushan Kumar**

Patient **Naveen Yadav** from **Faridabad** age **22 yrs** reported to N.I.C.E with the symptoms of **Fever, Sore throat, Headache, Body ache/muscle ache, Tiredness** on **06-Nov-20** got cured in **7 days** under the N.I.C.E Care of **Chotalia Sureshchandra**

Patient **Shrimanth Behere** from **Hyderabad** age **45 yrs** reported to N.I.C.E with the symptoms of **Fever, Sore throat, Body ache/muscle ache** on **23-Jun-20** got cured in **4 days** under the N.I.C.E Care of **Dr.Lakshminarayan Reddy**

Patient **Akash Jindal** from **Faridabad** age **29 yrs** reported to N.I.C.E with the symptoms of **Fever, Sore throat, Body ache/muscle ache, Tiredness, breathing difficulty** on **22-Jun-20** got cured in **7 days** under the N.I.C.E Care of **Dr Rajendra Prasad Kumawat**

Patient **Brij Mohan** from **New Delhi** age **34 yrs** reported to N.I.C.E with the symptoms of **Fever, Dry Cough, Headache, Tiredness** on **2-Jun-20** got cured in **6 days** under the N.I.C.E Care of **Chitra Jain**

Patient **Shubham Shivaji Randhe** from **Thane** age **23 yrs** reported to N.I.C.E with the symptoms of **Fever, Body ache/muscle ache** on **19-Jun-20** got cured in **8 days** under the N.I.C.E Care of **Rahul Bansal**

Patient **Ankur Singh** from **Ambedkar Nagar** age **21 yrs** reported to N.I.C.E with the symptoms of **Fever, Sore throat, Headache, Body ache/muscle ache, Tiredness** got cured in **3 days** under the N.I.C.E Care of **Rishu Garg**

Patient **Vinayak Patil** from **Navi Mumbai** age **32 yrs** reported to N.I.C.E with the symptoms of **Fever, Headache, Body ache/muscle**

ache, Tiredness on got cured in **4 days** under the N.I.C.E Care of **Ananta Kumar Panda**

Patient **Sumeet arora** from **New Delhi** age **45 yrs** reported to N.I.C.E with the symptoms of **Fever, Dry Cough, Headache, Body ache/muscle ache, Congestion, Tiredness** on **06-Nov-20** got cured in **8 days** under the N.I.C.E Care of **Rahul Bansal**

Patient **Rajesh Kumar** from **New delhi** age **48 yrs** reported to N.I.C.E with the symptoms of **Fever** got cured in **3 days** under the N.I.C.E Care of **Madhuri Anand Kinnikar**

Patient **VijayB Tambe** from **Thane** age **54 yrs** reported to N.I.C.E with the symptoms of **Fever, Sore throat, Body ache/muscle ache, breathing difficulty** on got cured in **3 days** under the N.I.C.E Care of **Bhagwan Dass**

Patient **Sheba t kurian** from **New Delhi** age **30 yrs** reported to N.I.C.E with the symptoms of **Sore throat, Headache, Tiredness** got cured in **3 days** under the N.I.C.E Care of **Raushan Kumar**

Patient **Shreepad** from **Mumbai** age **38 yrs** reported to N.I.C.E with the symptoms of **Fever, Body ache/muscle ache** on got cured in **3 days** under the N.I.C.E Care of **Raushan Kumar**

Patient **Akangsha Handique** from **Guwahati** age **6 yrs** reported to N.I.C.E with the symptoms of **Fever, Sore throat, Headache** on **12 Jun-20** got cured in **3 days** under the N.I.C.E Care of **Shikha Saxena**

Patient **Sagarmal jain** from **Navi mumbai** age **67 yrs** reported to N.I.C.E with the symptoms of **Fever, Dry Cough, Tiredness** on got cured in **2 days** under the N.I.C.E Care of **Dr Seema Arora**

Patient **Ritu** from **Noida** age **30 yrs** reported to N.I.C.E with the symptoms of **Fever, Dry Cough, Congestion** on **08-Jun-20** got cured in **3 days** under the N.I.C.E Care of **Mansi Thaker**

Patient **Neha Patel** from **Ahmedabad** age **30 yrs** reported to N.I.C.E with the symptoms of **Dry Cough, Sore throat** got cured in **2 days** under the N.I.C.E Care of **Suresh Kumar Yadav**

Patient **Naveen Panchal** from **Ahmedabad** age **46 yrs** reported to N.I.C.E with the symptoms of **Fever** got cured in **6 days** under the N.I.C.E Care of **Kanishk Amarpuri**

Patient **Devika thakur** from **Harda** age **30 yrs** reported to N.I.C.E with the symptoms of **Fever, Sore throat, Body ache/muscle ache, Tiredness, breathing difficulty** on **01-July-20** got cured in **3 days** under the N.I.C.E Care of **Raushan Kumar**

Patient **Arpit Dalwadi** from **Panvel** age **30 yrs** reported to N.I.C.E with the symptoms of **Headache, Tiredness,** got cured in **2 days** under the N.I.C.E Care of **Gaurav Jain**

Patient **Krishna kanojia** from **Meerut** age **22 yrs** reported to N.I.C.E with the symptoms of **Fever, Sore throat, Body ache/ muscle ache, Tiredness, breathing difficulty** got cured in **2 days** under the N.I.C.E Care of **Gaurav Jain**

Patient **Permendra Kumar** from **New Delhi** age **37 yrs** reported to N.I.C.E with the symptoms of **Sore throat, Headache, Body ache/ muscle ache** got cured in **1 days** under the N.I.C.E Care of **Gaurav Jain**

Patient **Gopal Kumar** from **Pathakhera** age **34 yrs** reported to N.I.C.E with the symptoms of **Dry Cough, Sore throat, Headache** got cured in **10 days** under the N.I.C.E Care of **Gaurav Jain**

Patient **Rajesh Jangid** from **Surat** age **54 yrs** reported to N.I.C.E with the symptoms of **breathing difficulty** got cured in **4 days** under the N.I.C.E Care of **Arun Kumar**

Patient **A Ray** from **Noida** age **40 yrs** reported to N.I.C.E with the symptoms of **Headache, Body ache/muscle ache, Tiredness, breathing difficulty** got cured in **17 days** under the N.I.C.E Care of **Sraban Baraik**

Patient **Ajoy Hazra** from **Kolkata** age **37 yrs** reported to N.I.C.E with the symptoms of **Dry Cough, Tiredness** on **01-Jul-20** got cured in **10 days** under the N.I.C.E Care of **Shaikh Warisha Nasim**

Patient **Chandulal** from **Hyderabad** age **50 yrs** reported to N.I.C.E with the symptoms of **Sore throat** got cured in **7 days** under the N.I.C.E Care of **Ekta singh**

Patient **Sneha Bahadur** from **Ghaziabad** age **46 yrs** reported to N.I.C.E with the symptoms of **Fever, Body ache/muscle ache, Tiredness** got cured in **6 days** under the N.I.C.E Care of **Ekta agarwal**

Patient **Vivek Parab** from **Thane** age **34 yrs** reported to N.I.C.E with the symptoms of **Fever, Dry Cough, Sore throat, breathing difficulty** got cured in **5 days** under the N.I.C.E Care of **Sushma Bengani**

Patient **Mahesh Sawant** from **Pune** age **42 yrs** reported to N.I.C.E with the symptoms of **Fever, Dry Cough, Sore throat, Headache, Congestion, breathing difficulty** got cured in **5 days** under the N.I.C.E Care of **Sushma Bengani**

Patient **Dipshita Chawla** from **New Delhi** age **13 yrs** reported to N.I.C.E with the symptoms of **Sore throat, Headache, Body ache/muscle ache, Tiredness** got cured in **2 days** under the N.I.C.E Care of **Ashish**

Patient **Kanchan** from **Thane** age **28 yrs** reported to N.I.C.E with the symptoms of **Fever, Sore throat, Headache, Body ache/muscle ache, Tiredness** got cured in **4 days** under the N.I.C.E Care of **Suman Chauhan**

Patient **Shubham Kumar Bunkar** from **Satna** age **22 yrs** reported to N.I.C.E with the symptoms of **Fever, Headache, breathing difficulty** got cured in **8 days** under the N.I.C.E Care of **Suman Chauhan**

Patient **Salman Ahmed** from **New Delhi** age **29 yrs** reported to N.I.C.E with the symptoms of **Dry Cough, Sore throat, Tiredness** on **11-Jun-20** got cured in **6 days** under the N.I.C.E Care of **Raushan Kumar**

Patient **N D Pancholi** from **Sahibabad** age **76 yrs** reported to N.I.C.E with the symptoms of **Fever, Dry Cough** got cured in **7 days** under the N.I.C.E Care of **Seema Manikkoth**

Patient **Prashant Vetam** from **Mumbai** age **37 yrs** reported to N.I.C.E with the symptoms of **Sore throat, Body ache/muscle ache** got cured in **4 days** under the N.I.C.E Care of **Sanjay Dhaduk**

Patient **Amarjeet Thapar** from **Mumbai** age **65 yrs** reported to N.I.C.E with the symptoms of **Fever, Sore throat, Body ache/muscle ache, Congestion, Tiredness** got cured in **3 days** under the N.I.C.E Care of **Geetika Kapoor**

Patient **Javed Akram** from **Malda** age **26 yrs** reported to N.I.C.E with the symptoms of **Fever, Dry Cough, Tiredness** got cured in **3 days** under the N.I.C.E Care of **Rupesh Kumar**

Patient **Saigopal Viyalla** from **Hyderabad** age **36 yrs** reported to N.I.C.E with the symptoms of **Tiredness, breathing difficulty** got cured in **2 days** under the N.I.C.E Care of **Avinash Popatrao Sabare**

Patient **sunit kumari** from **Darbhanga** age **54 yrs** reported to N.I.C.E with the symptoms of **Fever, Headache, Tiredness** got cured in **3 days** under the N.I.C.E Care of **Rupesh Kumar**

Patient **Omer bin ali** from **Hyderabad** age **34 yrs** reported to N.I.C.E with the symptoms of **Fever, Dry Cough, Headache, Body ache/muscle ache, Tiredness, breathing difficulty** got cured in **4 days** under the N.I.C.E Care of **Rahul Bansal**

Patient **Yogesh datar** from **Kalyan** age **35 yrs** reported to N.I.C.E with the symptoms of **Sore throat, breathing difficulty** got cured in **3 days** under the N.I.C.E Care of **Rahul Bansal**

Patient **Deepak** from **Baprola** age **41 yrs** reported to N.I.C.E with the symptoms of **Fever, Headache, Body ache/muscle ache** on **02-Jul-20** got cured in **3 days** under the N.I.C.E Care of **Amit Aneja**

Patient **Fareeha** from **Hyderabad** age **14 yrs** reported to N.I.C.E with the symptoms of **Dry Cough** on **03-Jul-20** got cured in **4 days** under the N.I.C.E Care of **Dr. Barin Kumar Roy**

Patient **Yogesh Kumar** from **Faridabad** age **35 yrs** reported to N.I.C.E with the symptoms of **Dry Cough, Body ache/muscle ache, Tiredness** on **03-Jul-20** got cured in **7 days** under the N.I.C.E Care of **Dr. Barin Kumar Roy**

Patient **R. S. Prasad** from **Vadodara** age **40 yrs** reported to N.I.C.E with the symptoms of **Fever, Headache, Body ache/muscle ache, Tiredness,** got cured in **3 days** under the N.I.C.E Care of **Dr. Barin Kumar Roy**

Patient **Arpit Khowal** from **New Delhi** age **22 yrs** reported to N.I.C.E with the symptoms of **Sore throat** got cured in **6 days** under the N.I.C.E Care of **Simi Handa**

Patient **Shameembanu** from **Hyderabad** age **33 yrs** reported to N.I.C.E with the symptoms of **breathing difficulty** got cured in **4 days** under the N.I.C.E Care of **Geetika kapoor**

Patient **Khairunnisa** from **Hyderabad** age **38 yrs** reported to N.I.C.E with the symptoms of **Tiredness** got cured in **7 days** under the N.I.C.E Care of **Satish Kumar Varma Vuppalapati**

Patient **Shila Bai Bhurewal** from **Jalna** age **34 yrs** reported to N.I.C.E with the symptoms of **Fever, Body ache/muscle ache/, Tiredness** on **06-Jul-20** got cured in **3 days** under the N.I.C.E Care of **Alisha Massey**

Patient **Ashok Kumar** from **New delhi** age **57 yrs** reported to N.I.C.E with the symptoms of **Fever, Body ache/muscle ache, Tiredness** got cured in **5 days** under the N.I.C.E Care of **Nishu Sandhya**

Patient **Birmla** from **Dwarka** age **59 yrs** reported to N.I.C.E with the symptoms of got cured in **3 days** under the N.I.C.E Care of **Nishu Sandhya**

Patient **Sanjay Gupta** from **New Delhi** age **40 yrs** reported to

N.I.C.E with the symptoms of **Dry Cough, Breathing difficulty** got cured in **7 days** under the N.I.C.E Care of **Nishu Sandhya**

Patient **Kannan Iyer** from **Mumbai** age **54 yrs** reported to N.I.C.E with the symptoms of **Fever, Headache, Body ache/muscle ache/, Tiredness Weakness** on **05-Jul-20** got cured in **9 days** under the N.I.C.E Care of **Ashish**

Patient **Athav Deshmukh** from **Akola** age **21 yrs** reported to N.I.C.E with the symptoms of **Dry Cough, breathing difficulty** got cured in **2 days** under the N.I.C.E Care of **Chotalia Sureshchandra**

Patient **Jaishree Jain** from **Ghaziabad** age **35 yrs** reported to N.I.C.E with the symptoms of **Fever, Headache** got cured in **8 days** under the N.I.C.E Care of **Deepti V Helgaonkar**

Patient **Mohd Sarwar** from **Hyderabad** age **37 yrs** reported to N.I.C.E with the symptoms of **Fever**

Headache, Body ache/muscle acheTiredness, Weakness on **09-Jul-20** got cured in **4 days** under the N.I.C.E Care of **Pragya Jha**

Patient **Mayur Rahul Bhaskar** from **Kalyan** age **28 yrs** reported to N.I.C.E with the symptoms of **Fever, Tiredness Weakness** on **06-Jul-20** got cured in **2 days** under the N.I.C.E Care of **Raushan Kumar**

Patient **Sawami** from **Naraina** age **36 yrs** reported to N.I.C.E with the symptoms of **Fever, Headache, Body ache/muscle ache/, Tiredness** on **05-Jul-20** got cured in **14 days** under the N.I.C.E Care of **Kimti Lal**

Patient **Yogita** from **Mumbai** age **42 yrs** reported to N.I.C.E with the symptoms of **Dry Cough, Sore throat, Headache, Body ache/ muscle ache, Tiredness** on **06-Jul-20** got cured in **4 days** under the N.I.C.E Care of **Najabhai Bhagvanbhai Chauhan**

Patient **Suneel kumar** from **New Delhi** age **26 yrs** reported to N.I.C.E with the symptoms of **Fever, Dry Cough, Sore throat,**

Headache, Tiredness, breathing difficulty on **09-Jul-20** got cured in **4 days** under the N.I.C.E Care of **Gopinath Narayanam**

Patient **Manik Lal Gupta** from **Lucknow** age **46 yrs** reported to N.I.C.E with the symptoms of **Fever, Sore throat, Tiredness, breathing difficulty** on **09-Jun-20** got cured in **15 days** under the N.I.C.E Care of **Poonam Arora**

Patient **Pradip Rathod** from **Ahmedabad** age **37 yrs** reported to N.I.C.E with the symptoms of **Fever, Tiredness** on **08-Jun-20** got cured in **2 days** under the N.I.C.E Care of **Anurag Mittal**

Patient **Sanved Rahul pawar** from **Shirwal** age **4 yrs** reported to N.I.C.E with the symptoms of **Fever** on **06-Oct-20** got cured in **2 days** under the N.I.C.E Care of **Dr. Narasinhaswami Mamdyal**

Patient **Sarabjeet Kaur** from **New Delhi** age **35 yrs** reported to N.I.C.E with the symptoms of **Fever, Dry Cough, Sore throat, Headache, Body ache/muscle ache, Tiredness** on **10-Jun-20** got cured in **3 days** under the N.I.C.E Care of **Ritesh Harshadkumar Chanpura**

Patient **Inderjeet Singh** from **New Delhi** age **63 yrs** reported to N.I.C.E with the symptoms of **Fever, Sore throat, Headache, Body ache/muscle ache, Tiredness, breathing difficulty** on **10-Jun-20** got cured in **10 days** under the N.I.C.E Care of **Subhas Mukherjee**

Patient **Rajbala** from **New Delhi** age **55 yrs** reported to N.I.C.E with the symptoms of **Fever, Dry Cough, Headache, Body ache/muscle ache** on **08-Jun-20** got cured in **7 days** under the N.I.C.E Care of **Rekha Gupta**

Patient **Deepanshu** from **New Delhi** age **25 yrs** reported to N.I.C.E with the symptoms of **Headache, Congestion, Tiredness** on **12-Jun-20** got cured in **3 days** under the N.I.C.E Care of **Bhupendra Singh Panwar**

Patient **Manmohan Singh** from **New Delhi** age **50 yrs** reported to N.I.C.E with the symptoms of **Fever, Sore throat, Headache, Body** ache/muscle ache on 08-Jun-20 got cured in 10 days under the N.I.C.E Care of **Kanishk Amarpuri**

Patient **Ashu** from **New Delhi** age **28 yrs** reported to N.I.C.E with the symptoms of **Fever, Dry Cough, Sore throat, Headache, Body ache/muscle ache, Tiredness** on 12-Jun-20 got cured in **3 days** under the N.I.C.E Care of **Filda Don**

Patient **Abhilekh Yadav** from **New Delhi** age **31 yrs** reported to N.I.C.E with the symptoms of **Sore throat** on 12-Jun-20 got cured in **3 days** under the N.I.C.E Care of **Rachna Sharma**

Patient **Aasma Khatoon** from **Kolkata** age **37 yrs** reported to N.I.C.E with the symptoms of **Fever** on 12-Jun-20 got cured in **4 days** under the N.I.C.E Care of **Kumar Shivam**

Patient **Ram Lakhan** from **New Delhi** age **63 yrs** reported to N.I.C.E with the symptoms of **Body ache/muscle ache, Tiredness, Breathing difficulty** got cured in **7 days** under the N.I.C.E Care of **Kalpana Bourai**

Patient **Santosh Kumar Mishra** from **New Delhi** age **44 yrs** reported to N.I.C.E with the symptoms of **Fever, Dry Cough, Sore throat, Tiredness** on 06-Dec-20 got cured in **15 days** under the N.I.C.E Care of **Dr. Narasinhaswami Mamdyal**

Patient **Shehzad Mulla** from **Baswan Bagewadi** age **42 yrs** reported to N.I.C.E with the symptoms of **Sore throat, Tiredness** got cured in **3 days** under the N.I.C.E Care of **Emmanuel Job**

Patient **Harmeet Singh** from **Ghaziabad** age **28 yrs** reported to N.I.C.E with the symptoms of **Fever, Tiredness** got cured in **2 days** under the N.I.C.E Care of **Chitra Jain**

Patient **Rajni** from **Gurugram** age **35 yrs** reported to N.I.C.E with the symptoms of **Sore throat** got cured in **2 days** under the N.I.C.E Care of **Rachna Sharma**

Patient **Gajender Singh** from **New Delhi** age **36 yrs** reported to N.I.C.E with the symptoms of **Sore throat, Headache, Body ache/**

muscle ache, Congestion, breathing difficulty got cured in **4 days** under the N.I.C.E Care of **Kalpana Bourai**

Patient **Ranjit kumar giri** from **Jalandhar** age **38 yrs** reported to N.I.C.E with the symptoms of **Sore throat, Congestion** on 12-Jun-20 got cured in **10 days** under the N.I.C.E Care of **Emmanuel Job**

Patient **Varsha Sharma** from **Khera khurd** age **22 yrs** reported to N.I.C.E with the symptoms of **Dry Cough, Sore throat, Headache, Body ache/muscle ache, Tiredness** got cured in **7 days** under the N.I.C.E Care of **Pratiksha Vats**

Patient **Rakesh kumar** from **Chandigarh** age **10 yrs** reported to N.I.C.E with the symptoms of **Fever** got cured in **3 days** under the N.I.C.E Care of **Sourav Bysack**

Patient **Raghav** from **Chandigarh** age **10 yrs** reported to N.I.C.E with the symptoms of **Fever** got cured in **2 days** under the N.I.C.E Care of **Sourav Bysack**

Patient **Sagar Ahiwale** from age **23 yrs** reported to N.I.C.E with the symptoms of **Dry Cough, Sore throat, Headache, Tiredness, breathing difficulty** on **02-Jun-20** got cured in **2 days** under the N.I.C.E Care of **Emmanuel Job**

Patient **Ramesh Chand** from **New Delhi** age **54 yrs** reported to N.I.C.E with the symptoms of **Fever, Dry Cough** got cured in **2 days** under the N.I.C.E Care of **Amit Aneja**

Patient **Avtar singh** from **New Delhi** age **48 yrs** reported to N.I.C.E with the symptoms of **Fever, Body ache/muscle ache** got cured in **7 days** under the N.I.C.E Care of **Rameshwar Thokchom**

Patient **Sunil** from **Sangamner** age **41 yrs** reported to N.I.C.E with the symptoms of **Dry Cough, Sore throat** got cured in **10 days** under the N.I.C.E Care of **Rachna Sharma**

Patient **Afreen Badgujar** from **Hyderabad** age **27 yrs** reported to N.I.C.E with the suspected symptoms of influenza got cured in **7 days** under the N.I.C.E Care of **Pratiksha Vats**

Patient **Paresh Kori** from **Mumbai** age **19 yrs** reported to N.I.C.E with the symptoms of **Fever, Sore throat, Body ache/muscle ache** got cured in **4 days** under the N.I.C.E Care of **Raj Kishore Kodwani**

Patient **Agha Arshi Mirza** from **Varanasi** age **40 yrs** reported to N.I.C.E with the symptoms of **Dry Cough, Body ache/muscle ache, Tiredness, breathing difficulty** got cured in **9 days** under the N.I.C.E Care of **Kalpana Bourai**

Patient **Sunita Devi** from **West Vinod Nagar** age **45 yrs** reported to N.I.C.E with the symptoms of **Dry Cough, Sore throat, Breathing difficulty** got cured in **5 days** under the N.I.C.E Care of **Rachna Sharma**

Patient **Gopal** from **Sonipat** age **34 yrs** reported to N.I.C.E with the symptoms of **Fever, Sore throat, Headache, Body ache/muscle ache, Tiredness** got cured in **3 days** under the N.I.C.E Care of **Adarsha Narayan Pradhan**

Patient **Goutam Halwa** from **Nawrangpur** age **32 yrs** reported to N.I.C.E with the symptoms of **Dry Cough, Tiredness** got cured in **12 days** under the N.I.C.E Care of **Pratiksha Vats**

Patient **Chetna** from **New Delhi** age **23 yrs** reported to N.I.C.E with the symptoms of **Dry Cough, Tiredness,** on **06-Nov-20** got cured in **2 days** under the N.I.C.E Care of **Kalpana Bourai**

Patient **Sumit Goyal** from **Ajmer** age **33 yrs** reported to N.I.C.E with the symptoms of **Dry Cough** got cured in **15 days** under the N.I.C.E Care of **Rachna Sharma**

Patient **Vikash Saha** from **Dhanbad** age **28 yrs** reported to N.I.C.E with the symptoms of **Headache,** got cured in **3 days** under the N.I.C.E Care of **Pratiksha Vats**

Patient **Nirmal Debnath** from **Mumbai** age **49 yrs** reported to N.I.C.E with the symptoms of **Sore throat** got cured in **3 days** under the N.I.C.E Care of **Kalpana Bourai**

Patient **Rahulb Kamble** from **Thane** age **44 yrs** reported to N.I.C.E with the symptoms of **Fever, Headache, Body ache/muscle ache, Tiredness** got cured in **3 days** under the N.I.C.E Care of **Rajendra Patil**

Patient **Birendra Dutta** from **Mumbai** age **39 yrs** reported to N.I.C.E with the symptoms of **Dry Cough, Sore throat, Congestion** on **05-Jun-20** got cured in **10 days** under the N.I.C.E Care of **Emmanuel Job**

Patient **Himanshu** from **Sherkot** age **31 yrs** reported to N.I.C.E with the symptoms of **Body ache/muscle ache, breathing difficulty** got cured in **15 days** under the N.I.C.E Care of **Rachna Sharma**

Patient **Anil Kumar Gupta** from **North 24 Parganas** age **57 yrs** reported to N.I.C.E with the symptoms of **Fever, Tiredness** got cured in **3 days** under the N.I.C.E Care of **Seema Manikkoth**

Patient **Surrender Pal Singh** from **New Delhi** age **53 yrs** reported to N.I.C.E with the symptoms of **Dry Cough, breathing difficulty** got cured in **3 days** under the N.I.C.E Care of **Pratiksha Vats**

Patient **Shishupal** from **Kekri** age **24 yrs** reported to N.I.C.E with the symptoms of **Sore throat, Body ache/muscle ache, Tiredness** got cured in **6 days** under the N.I.C.E Care of **Kalpana Bourai**

Patient **Sanjay kumar** from **Kosi Kalan** age **40 yrs** reported to N.I.C.E with the symptoms of **Dry Cough, Sore throat, Headache, Body ache/muscle ache, Congestion, Tiredness** got cured in **3 days** under the N.I.C.E Care of **Emmanuel Job**

Patient **Laxmi Sharma** from **New Delhi** age **47 yrs** reported to N.I.C.E with the symptoms of **Fever, Dry Cough, Headache** got cured in **3 days** under the N.I.C.E Care of **Amrut Tikamchand Singhavi**

Patient **Avinash Tayade** from **Savada** age **25 yrs** reported to N.I.C.E with the symptoms of **Headache, Body ache/muscle ache, Tiredness, breathing difficulty** got cured in **3 days** under the N.I.C.E Care of **Rachna Sharma**

Patient **Srujana** from **Santhanutala Padu** age **40 yrs** reported to N.I.C.E with the symptoms of **Dry Cough, Body ache/muscle ache, breathing difficulty** got cured in **2 days** under the N.I.C.E Care of **Pratiksha Vats**

Patient **Tushar** from **New Delhi** age **41 yrs** reported to N.I.C.E with the symptoms of **Fever** on **12-Jun-20** got cured in **7 days** under the N.I.C.E Care of **Adv Syed Wajid Husain**

Patient **Roshni Devi** from **Gurugram** age **30 yrs** reported to N.I.C.E with the symptoms of **Dry Cough, Sore throat, Headache, Body ache/muscle ache, Tiredness** got cured in **5 days** under the N.I.C.E Care of **Kalpana Bourai**

Patient **Aryan** from **New Delhi** age **18 yrs** reported to N.I.C.E with the symptoms of **Fever, Dry Cough, Sore throat, breathing difficulty** got cured in **12 days** under the N.I.C.E Care of **Kavitha N Jain**

Patient **Omar Shaikh** from **Solapur** age **31 yrs** reported to N.I.C.E with the symptoms of **Fever, Body ache/muscle ache, Congestion, Tiredness** got cured in **3 days** under the N.I.C.E Care of **Sanjay Gupta**

Patient **Arun Surana** from **New Delhi** age **65 yrs** reported to N.I.C.E with the symptoms of **Body ache/muscle ache, Tiredness** got cured in **10 days** under the N.I.C.E Care of **Emmanuel Job**

Patient **Narinder** from **New Delhi** age **65 yrs** reported to N.I.C.E with the symptoms of **Fever** got cured in **1 days** under the N.I.C.E Care of **Dr. Atul Ramesh Narkhede**

Patient **Sharang S Sankpal** from **Mumbai** age **40 yrs** reported to N.I.C.E with the symptoms of **Sore throat** got cured in **3 days** under the N.I.C.E Care of **Rachna Sharma**

Patient **Pratibha** from **New Delhi** age **26 yrs** reported to N.I.C.E with the symptoms of **Dry Cough, Sore throat, Headache, Tiredness** got cured in **4 days** under the N.I.C.E Care of **Kalpana Bourai**

Patient **Sujan Sunar** from **Jalpaiguri** age **27 yrs** reported to N.I.C.E with the symptoms of **Headache, Tiredness, Breathing difficulty** got cured in **4 days** under the N.I.C.E Care of **Emmanuel Job**

Patient **Divyam Bhakuni** from **Ghaziabad** age **17 yrs** reported to N.I.C.E with the symptoms of **Fever, Dry Cough, Headache** got cured in **5 days** under the N.I.C.E Care of **Nishu Sandhya**

Patient **Kalyani** from **Jaipur** age **28 yrs** reported to N.I.C.E with the symptoms of **Headache, Body ache/muscle ache, Tiredness** got cured in **4 days** under the N.I.C.E Care of **Hulash Chand Sankhla**

Patient **Arpit Sachan** from **Jhansi** age **23 yrs** reported to N.I.C.E with the symptoms of **breathing difficulty** got cured in **3 days** under the N.I.C.E Care of **Rachna Sharma**

Patient **Krishna Datta Pandit** from **Nagpur** age **33 yrs** reported to N.I.C.E with the symptoms of **Headache, Body ache/muscle ache** got cured in **3 days** under the N.I.C.E Care of **Pratiksha Vats**

Patient **Manisha Toshniwal** from **Hyderabad** age **29 yrs** reported to N.I.C.E with the symptoms of **Headache, Body ache/muscle ache** got cured in **4 days** under the N.I.C.E Care of **Kalpana Bourai**

Patient **Saurabh Singh Tomar** from **Bhiwadi** age **22 yrs** reported to N.I.C.E with the symptoms of **Dry Cough, Congestion** got cured in **11 days** under the N.I.C.E Care of **Emmanuel Job**

Patient **Brindaban Mandal** from **Jhargram** age **33 yrs** reported to N.I.C.E with the symptoms of **Fever, Dry Cough, Tiredness** got cured in **2 days** under the N.I.C.E Care of **Amit Aneja**

Patient **Suman Khan** from **Arambagh** age **23 yrs** reported to N.I.C.E with the symptoms of **Sore throat** on **18-Jun-20** got cured in **3 days** under the N.I.C.E Care of **Lomash Anand**

Patient **Sudarshan** from **Bengaluru** age **42 yrs** reported to N.I.C.E with the symptoms of **Fever, Dry Cough, Body ache/muscle ache, Tiredness** on **30-Jun-20** got cured in **5 days** under the N.I.C.E Care of **Ashok N Adak**

Patient **Hariom Sharma** from **New Delhi** age **36 yrs** reported to N.I.C.E with the symptoms of **Dry Cough, breathing difficulty** on **25-Jun-20** got cured in **7 days** under the N.I.C.E Care of **Ashok N Adak**

Patient **Vidyasagar** from **Arrah** age **26 yrs** reported to N.I.C.E with the symptoms of **Dry Cough** got cured in **3 days** under the N.I.C.E Care of **Lomash Anand**

Patient **Narender Kumar** from **New Delhi** age **46 yrs** reported to N.I.C.E with the symptoms of **Fever, Sore throat, Headache, Body ache/muscle ache, Tiredness** on **16-Jun-20** got cured in **5 days** under the N.I.C.E Care of **Bhatkar**

Patient **Kunal Mohan Chavhan** from **Bhiwandi** age **23 yrs** reported to N.I.C.E with the symptoms of **Dry Cough, Tiredness** on **26-Jun-20** got cured in **7 days** under the N.I.C.E Care of **Dr Rajendra Prasad Kumawat**

Patient **Kaptan** from **Delhi** age **62 yrs** reported to N.I.C.E with the symptoms of **Fever, Headache, Body ache/muscle ache, Tiredness** on **27-Jun-20** got cured in **7 days** under the N.I.C.E Care of **Adarsha Narayan Pradhan**

Patient **Ritesh** from **Bikaner** age **20 yrs** reported to N.I.C.E with the symptoms of **Fever** on **15-Jun-20** got cured in **4 days** under the N.I.C.E Care of **Ayan Haldar**

Patient **Vikas Sardesai** from **Pune** age **33 yrs** reported to N.I.C.E with the symptoms of **Fever, Weakness** on **08-Jul-20** got cured in **5 days** under the N.I.C.E Care of **Pragya Jha**

Patient **Shailesh** from **Ambernath** age **29 yrs** reported to N.I.C.E with the symptoms of **Fever, Dry Cough, Body ache/muscle ache/, Tiredness Weakness** on **06-Jul-20** got cured in **5 days** under the N.I.C.E Care of **Kapil Dev Sharma**

Patient **Preethi** from **Hanumanthnagar** age **33 yrs** reported to N.I.C.E with the symptoms of **Headache, Tiredness Weakness** got cured in **5 days** under the N.I.C.E Care of **Kapil Dev Sharma**

Patient **Chandan Kumar Nirala** from **Bhagalpur** age **35 yrs** reported to N.I.C.E with the symptoms of **Fever, Dry Cough, Headache, Body ache/muscle ache** got cured in **4 days** under the N.I.C.E Care of **Kapil Dev Sharma**

Patient **Ashish Jaiswal** from **Chennai** age **40 yrs** reported to N.I.C.E with the symptoms of **Fever, Dry Cough, breathing difficulty** got cured in **7 days** under the N.I.C.E Care of **deepti v helgaonkar**

Patient **Kumari Jyothi** from **Gwalior** age **32 yrs** reported to N.I.C.E with the symptoms of **Dry Cough, Congestion, Tiredness Weakness** on **05-Jul-20** got cured in **4 days** under the N.I.C.E Care of **Preethi Katariya**

Patient **Mohd Aslam** from **Kannauj** age **26 yrs** reported to N.I.C.E with the symptoms of **breathing difficulty** on **01-Jul-20** got cured in **7 days** under the N.I.C.E Care of **Rahul Bansal**

Patient **Abhishek Mishra** from **New Delhi** age **23 yrs** reported to N.I.C.E with the symptoms of **Fever, Headache, Body ache/muscle ache/, Tiredness Weakness** on **07-Jul-20** got cured in **3 days** under the N.I.C.E Care of **Suresh Kumar Yadav**

Patient **Lokesh Sharma** from **Greater Noida** age **27 yrs** reported to N.I.C.E with the symptoms of **Fever, Tiredness Weakness** on **06-Jul-20** got cured in **5 days** under the N.I.C.E Care of **Raushan Kumar**

Patient **Suleman Khan** from **D** age **25 yrs** reported to N.I.C.E with the symptoms of **Fever, Body ache/muscle ache/, Tiredness Weakness** on **06-Jul-20** got cured in **4 days** under the N.I.C.E Care of **Dr.Sheetal Nimkande**

Patient **Ashish Sharma** from **Mumbai** age **39 yrs** reported to N.I.C.E with the symptoms of **Fever, Tiredness Weakness** on **28-May-20** got cured in **4 days** under the N.I.C.E Care of **Dharmendra Kumar Pandey**

Patient **Ayushman Dey** from **Kolkata** age **7 yrs** reported to N.I.C.E with the symptoms of **Fever, Body ache/muscle ache/, Weakness** on **08-Jul-20** got cured in **3 days** under the N.I.C.E Care of **Dharmendra Kumar Pandey**

Patient **Mukesh Bhagat** from **Bardoli** age **60 yrs** reported to N.I.C.E with the suspected symptoms of influenza on **10-Jul-20** got cured in **3 days** under the N.I.C.E Care of **Ekta Agarwal**

Patient **Varun siotia** from **Chennai** age **20 yrs** reported to N.I.C.E with the symptoms of **Headache, Tiredness , Weakness** on **10-Jul-20** got cured in **6 days** under the N.I.C.E Care of **Ekta Agarwal**

Patient **Dipankar Dash** from **Gurugram** age **30 yrs** reported to N.I.C.E with the symptoms of **Fever, Sore throat, Headache, Body ache/muscle ache/, Tiredness Weakness** on **07-Jul-20** got cured in **3 days** under the N.I.C.E Care of **Bhagwan Dass**

Patient **G.Shaikh** from **Pune** age **39 yrs** reported to N.I.C.E with the symptoms of **Fever, Dry Cough, Body ache/muscle ache/, Tiredness Weakness** on **25-Jun-20** got cured in **4 days** under the N.I.C.E Care of **Sayed Shah**

Patient **Vinod** from **Akbarpur** age **28 yrs** reported to N.I.C.E with the symptoms of **Fever, Sore throat, Congestion, Tiredness** on **07-Jul-20** got cured in **3 days** under the N.I.C.E Care of **Sayed Shah**

Patient **Sangeeta** from **Faridabad** age **31 yrs** reported to N.I.C.E with the symptoms of **Dry Cough, Headache, Body ache/muscle ache, Tiredness** on **17-Jun-20** got cured in **3 days** under the N.I.C.E Care of **Arvind Kumar Plaha**

Patient **Baljeet Kaur** from **Torrejon de ardoz** age **37 yrs** reported to N.I.C.E with the symptoms of **Fever, Breathing difficulty, Weakness** on **07-Jun-20** got cured in **5 days** under the N.I.C.E Care of **Simi Handa**

Patient **Shiver Das** from **Kolkata** age **49 yrs** reported to N.I.C.E with the symptoms of **Fever** on **08-Jul-20** got cured in **6 days** under the N.I.C.E Care of **Arvind Kumar Plaha**

Patient **Dinesh Kumar** from **New Delhi** age 45 yrs reported to N.I.C.E with the symptoms of **Fever, breathing difficulty** on 08-**Jul-20** got cured in **4 days** under the N.I.C.E Care of **Arvind Kumar Plaha**

Patient **Vaishali Verma** from **Mumbai** age **43 yrs** reported to N.I.C.E with the symptoms of **Fever, Congestion, breathing difficulty** on **08-Jul-20** got cured in **6 days** under the N.I.C.E Care of **Arvind Kumar Plaha**

Patient **Tarun Arora** from **New Delhi** age **37 yrs** reported to N.I.C.E with the symptoms of **Sore throat, Headache, Body ache/muscle ache/, Tiredness Weakness** on **10-Jul-20** got cured in **3 days** under the N.I.C.E Care of **Ekta agarwal**

Patient **Yogesh Chahar** from **Mahoba** age **27 yrs** reported to N.I.C.E with the symptoms of **Dry Cough, Sore throat, Headache, Body ache/muscle ache/, Tiredness Breathing difficulty, Weakness** on **06-Jul-20** got cured in **4 days** under the N.I.C.E Care of **Brijmohan Yadav**

Patient **Md Hasnain Ansari** from **Kolkata** age **4 yrs** reported to N.I.C.E with the symptoms of **Fever, Weakness** on **10-Jul-20** got cured in **3 days** under the N.I.C.E Care of **Brijmohan Yadav**

Patient **Vima** from **Degam** age **45 yrs** reported to N.I.C.E with the symptoms of **Headache** on **03-Jul-20** got cured in **3 days** under the N.I.C.E Care of **Goma Ram**

Patient **Ankahi N Jain** from **Mumbai** age **15 yrs** reported to N.I.C.E with the symptoms of **Fever, Headache, Body ache/muscle ache/, Tiredness Weakness** on **08-Jul-20** got cured in **5 days** under the N.I.C.E Care of **Kamal Dhawan**

Patient **Javed Khan** from **Mumbai** age **40 yrs** reported to N.I.C.E with the symptoms of **Fever, Congestion** on **07-Jul-20** got cured in **5 days** under the N.I.C.E Care of **Suresh Kumar Yadav**

Patient **Chander Mohan** from **New Delhi** age **46 yrs** reported to N.I.C.E with the symptoms of **Fever, Headache, Body ache/muscle** ache/, Tiredness Weakness on 07-Jul-20 got cured in 5 days under the N.I.C.E Care of Dr Puran Sharma

Patient Bittu from New Delhi age 30 yrs reported to N.I.C.E with the symptoms of Fever, Dry Cough, Sore throat, Headache, Body ache/muscle ache/, Congestion, Tiredness Weakness on 05-Jul-20 got cured in 3 days under the N.I.C.E Care of Dr Puran Sharma

Patient Vasudev Bhat from Hyderabad age 34 yrs reported to N.I.C.E with the symptoms of Fever on 07-Jul-20 got cured in 7 days under the N.I.C.E Care of Dr Puran Sharma

Patient Kumari Sudha from Khagaria age 35 yrs reported to N.I.C.E with the symptoms of Fever, Sore throat, Body ache/muscle ache/, Congestion, Tiredness breathing difficulty, Weakness on 07-Jul-20 got cured in 4 days under the N.I.C.E Care of suresh Kumar Yadav

Patient Basavaraj patil from Panvel age 32 yrs reported to N.I.C.E with the symptoms of Fever on 05-Jul-20 got cured in 6 days under the N.I.C.E Care of Kimti Lal

Patient Mandar Shahasnr from Badlapur west age 46 yrs reported to N.I.C.E with the symptoms of Fever on 12-Jul-20 got cured in 5 days under the N.I.C.E Care of Shiv Dular

Patient Md. Nizamuddin from Raxaul age 50 yrs reported to N.I.C.E with the symptoms of Dry Cough, Congestion, breathing difficulty, Weakness on 07-Jul-20 got cured in 7 days under the N.I.C.E Care of Sraban Baraik

Patient Saksham from Bengaluru age 16 yrs reported to N.I.C.E with the symptoms of Fever got cured in 5 days under the N.I.C.E Care of Dr. Kishan Pareek

Patient Neelu Jaiswal from North 24 Parganas age 42 yrs reported to N.I.C.E with the symptoms of Fever, Body ache/muscle ache/, Weakness on 08-Jul-20 got cured in 7 days under the N.I.C.E Care of Dr. Kishan Pareek

Patient **Deepinder Kaur** from **Phagwara/ jalandhar** age **27 yrs** reported to N.I.C.E with the symptoms of **Fever, Sore throat, Tiredness** on **01-Jul-20** got cured in **3 days** under the N.I.C.E Care of **Chitra Jain**

Patient **Sweta singhi** from **Kolkata** age **57 yrs** reported to N.I.C.E with the symptoms of **Fever, Dry Cough, Sore throat, Headache, Body ache/muscle ache/, Tiredness Weakness** on **07-Jul-20** got cured in **6 days** under the N.I.C.E Care of **Dushyant Chaturvedi**

Patient **Rakesh** from **Bengaluru** age **32 yrs** reported to N.I.C.E with the symptoms of **Sore throat** on **11-Jul-20** got cured in **6 days** under the N.I.C.E Care of **Dr Seema Arora**

Patient **Vishal Pingle** from **Thane** age **34 yrs** reported to N.I.C.E with the symptoms of **Fever, Headache, Weakness** on **26-Jun-20** got cured in **5 days** under the N.I.C.E Care of **Dr Seema Arora**

Patient **Shivraj Thorat** from **Manchar** age **24 yrs** reported to N.I.C.E with the symptoms of **Dry Cough, Tiredness** on **12-Jul-20** got cured in **4 days** under the N.I.C.E Care of **Nishu Sandhya**

Patient **P. Rajender Ready** from **Hyderabad** age **35 yrs** reported to N.I.C.E with the symptoms of **Fever, Weakness** on **08-Jul-20** got cured in **4 days** under the N.I.C.E Care of **Goma Ram**

Patient **Neeraj Sharma** from **New Delhi** age **30 yrs** reported to N.I.C.E with the symptoms of **Sore throat, breathing difficulty** on **19-Jun-20** got cured in **5 days** under the N.I.C.E Care of **Ekta Agarwal**

Patient **Chintan Shah** from **Surat** age **31 yrs** reported to N.I.C.E with the symptoms of **Fever, Sore throat, Body ache/muscle ache/, Tiredness Weakness** on **07-Jul-20** got cured in **4 days** under the N.I.C.E Care of **Nishan Singh Jamwal**

Patient **Indu Shetty** from **Kolkata** age **42 yrs** reported to N.I.C.E with the symptoms of **Fever, Body ache/muscle ache/** on **09-Jul-20** got cured in **7 days** under the N.I.C.E Care of **Renu Garg**

Patient **Yash** from **Ahmedabad** age **22 yrs** reported to N.I.C.E with the symptoms of **Sore throat, Body ache/muscle ache/, Congestion, Tiredness Weakness** on **08-Jul-20** got cured in **6 days** under the N.I.C.E Care of **Samir Das**

Patient **Arushi Jain** from **Ludhiana** age **23 yrs** reported to N.I.C.E with the symptoms of **Fever, Dry Cough, Sore throat, Body ache/ Muscle ache/, Tiredness Weakness** on **11-Jul-20** got cured in **6 days** under the N.I.C.E Care of **Kavitha N Jain**

Patient **Sagar Somnath Dhikale** from **Badlapur west** age **33 yrs** reported to N.I.C.E with the symptoms of **Fever, Dry Cough, Headache, Tiredness** on **22-Jun-20** got cured in **7 days** under the N.I.C.E Care of **Kavitha N Jain**

Patient **Prashant J Patil** from **Kalyan** age **38 yrs** reported to N.I.C.E with the symptoms of **Fever, Headache, Body ache/muscle ache/, Weakness** on **10-Jul-20** got cured in **4 days** under the N.I.C.E Care of **Rameshwar Thokchom**

Patient **Harish Jadhav** from **Thane** age **59 yrs** reported to N.I.C.E with the symptoms of **Fever** on **12-Jul-20** got cured in **7 days** under the N.I.C.E Care of **Ashok N Adak**

Patient **Sunit Ghosh** from **Thane** age **28 yrs** reported to N.I.C.E with the symptoms of **breathing difficulty** on **10-Jul-20** got cured in **7 days** under the N.I.C.E Care of **Kapil Dev Sharma**

Patient **Dr kaushal** from **Ahmedabad** age **44 yrs** reported to N.I.C.E with the symptoms of **Fever, Headache, Body ache/muscle ache/, Tiredness Weakness** on **26-Jul-76** got cured in **4 days** under the N.I.C.E Care of **Raushan Kumar**

Patient **Sagar Somnath Dhikale** from **Badlapur west** age **33 yrs** reported to N.I.C.E with the symptoms of **Fever, Dry Cough, Headache, Tiredness** on **22-Jun-20** got cured in **5 days** under the N.I.C.E Care of **Kavitha N Jain**

Patient **Harshal Kharat** from **Ulhasnagar** age **32 yrs** reported to N.I.C.E with the symptoms of **Fever, Headache, Body ache/muscle** ache/, **Tiredness** on **10-Jul-20** got cured in **4 days** under the N.I.C.E Care of **Kamlakshi Shahdeo**

Patient **Sunil** from **Noida** age **35 yrs** reported to N.I.C.E with the symptoms of **Headache, Body ache/muscle ache/, Tiredness Weakness** on **04-Jul-20** got cured in **6 days** under the N.I.C.E Care of **Rajeev Kumar**

Patient **Karan Lakhee.** from **Sonepat** age **26 yrs** reported to N.I.C.E with the symptoms of **Body ache/muscle ache/, Tiredness Weakness** on **07-Jul-94** got cured in **5 days** under the N.I.C.E Care of **Bhagwan Dass**

Patient **Rina Jignesh Vora** from **surat** age **30 yrs** reported to N.I.C.E with the symptoms of **Congestion, Tiredness, breathing difficulty, Weakness** got cured in **5 days** under the N.I.C.E Care of **Bhagwan Dass**

Patient **Subham Ram Panchadane** from **Aurangabad** age **23 yrs** reported to N.I.C.E with the symptoms of **Fever, Dry Cough, Body ache/muscle ache/, Congestion** on **11-Jul-20** got cured in **7 days** under the N.I.C.E Care of **Bhagwan Dass**

Patient **Amit** from **Pune** age **23 yrs** reported to N.I.C.E with the symptoms of **Fever, Sore throat, Tiredness, Weakness** on **13-Jul-20** got cured in **6 days** under the N.I.C.E Care of **Nishu Sandhya**

Patient **Manish Kumar Patel** from **Surat** age **40 yrs** reported to N.I.C.E with the symptoms of **Headache, Congestion, Tiredness** on **12-Jul-20** got cured in **4 days** under the N.I.C.E Care of **Nishu Sandhya**

Patient **Navnath Rogade** from **Udgir** age **35 yrs** reported to N.I.C.E with the symptoms of **Fever, Sore throat, Body ache/muscle ache, Tiredness, Weakness** on **12-Jul-20** got cured in **7 days** under the N.I.C.E Care of **Nishu Sandhya**

Patient **Nupur Sharma** from *Surat* age **33 yrs** reported to N.I.C.E with the symptoms of **Fever, Dry Cough, Headache, Body ache/**

muscle ache, **Tiredness** on **25-Jun-20** with comorbidities like **Hypothyroidism, Rheumatic fever** got cured in **5 days** under the N.I.C.E Care of **Gopinath Narayanam**

Patient **Sayed abdullah** from *Darbhanga* age 34 yrs reported to N.I.C.E with the symptoms of **Dry Cough, Sore throat, Headache, Body ache/muscle ache/, Tiredness, Weakness** on **06-Jul-20** with comorbidity like **Diabetes** got cured in **4 days** under the N.I.C.E Care of **Milesh Sahare**

Patient **Rahul Jain** from *Hiriyur* age 20 yrs reported to N.I.C.E with the symptoms of **Fever, Body ache/muscle ache/, Weakness** on **08-Jul-20** with comorbidity like **Allergic rhinitis** got cured in **4 days** under the N.I.C.E Care of **Sounak Das**

Patient **Praveen** from *New Delhi* age 47 yrs reported to N.I.C.E with the symptoms of **Fever, Sore throat** on **16-Jun-20** with comorbidity like **Diabetes** got cured in **3 days** under the N.I.C.E Care of **Nilima Bhatkar**

Patient **Mrs. Krishna Paul** from *New Delhi* age 77 yrs reported to N.I.C.E with the symptoms of **Fever, Body ache/muscle ache, Tiredness** on **20-Jun-20** with comorbidities like **Hypertension, Diabetes** got cured in **4 days** under the N.I.C.E Care of **Prabhjot Kaur**

Patient **Dr Trilochan jena** from *Bhanjanagar* age 42 yrs reported to N.I.C.E with the symptoms of **Dry Cough, Sore throat** on **04-Jul-20** with comorbidity like **Spondylitis** got cured in **3 days** under the N.I.C.E Care of **Nishu Sandhya**

Patient **Jitendra Narayan Sharma** from *Varanasi* age **65 yrs** reported to N.I.C.E with the symptoms of **Fever, Dry Cough** on **06-Nov-20** with comorbidity like **Diabetes** got cured in **7 days** under the N.I.C.E Care of **Iqra Shaikh**

Patient **GP Sharma** from *Gurugram* age 55 yrs reported to N.I.C.E with the symptoms of **Fever, Dry Cough, breathing difficulty** on **06-Nov-20** with comorbidity like **Diabetes** got cured in **7 days** under the N.I.C.E Care of **Rishu Garg**

Patient **Devika Bhandare** from *Ambernath* age **45 yrs** reported to N.I.C.E with the symptoms of **Fever, Dry Cough, Sore throat, Body ache/muscle ache, Tiredness** with comorbidity like **Diabetes** got cured in **2 days** under the N.I.C.E Care of **Kanishk Amarpuri**

Patient **Mahendra Singh** from *Mumbai* age **55 yrs** reported to N.I.C.E with the symptom of **Fever** with comorbidity like **Diabetes** got cured in **2 days** under the N.I.C.E Care of **Chotalia Sureshchandra**

Patient **Satyapal** from *New Delhi* age **65 yrs** reported to N.I.C.E with the symptoms of **Fever, Dry Cough, Sore throat, Tiredness, breathing difficulty** with comorbidities like **Diabetes, hypertension** got cured in **5 days** under the N.I.C.E Care of **Reena Thakur**

Patient **Mushtaq Ahmed** from *Bengaluru* age **37 yrs** reported to N.I.C.E with the symptom of **Fever** with comorbidities like **Hypertension** got cured in **3 days** under the N.I.C.E Care of **Shaikh Warisha Nasim**

Patient **Tilak Chawla** from *Faridabad* age **42 yrs** reported to N.I.C.E with the symptoms of **Fever, Sore throat, Headache, Body ache/muscle ache, Congestion, Tiredness** on **11-Jun-20** with comorbidity like **IBS** got cured in **10 days** under the N.I.C.E Care of **Siddhartha Jain**

Patient **Rajalinga Reddy** from *Secundarabad* age **37 yrs** reported to N.I.C.E with the symptom of **Fever** with comorbidity like **Kidney Stones** got cured in **7 days** under the N.I.C.E Care of **Kanishk Amarpuri**

Patient **Ram Lakhan** from *New Delhi* age **54 yrs** reported to N.I.C.E with the symptoms of **Fever, Body ache/muscle ache, Tiredness** and comorbidity like **Hypertension** got cured in **3 days** under the N.I.C.E Care of **Shikha Saxena**

Patient **Viraj Dogra** from *New Delhi* age **50 yrs** reported to N.I.C.E with the symptoms of **Fever, Sore throat** with comorbidity like **Diabetes** got cured in **9 days** under the N.I.C.E Care of **Ajit Kumar Burnwal**

Patient **Sumeet** from *Gurugram* age **44 yrs** reported to N.I.C.E with suspected influenza and comorbidity like **Diabetes** got cured in **14 days** under the N.I.C.E Care of **Ashish**

Patient **Nanu ram sharma** from *New Delhi* age **64 yrs** reported to N.I.C.E with the symptoms of **Fever, Dry Cough** with comorbidities like **Hypertension, Diabetes, Heart disease** got cured in **14 days** under the N.I.C.E Care of **Ashish**

Patient **Anokh Vohra** from *Amritsar* age **65 yrs** reported to N.I.C.E with the symptoms of **Sore throat, Headache, Body ache/ muscle ache, Congestion, Tiredness, breathing difficulty** with comorbidity like **Ulcer** got cured in **3 days** under the N.I.C.E Care of **Ashish**

Patient **Arzana** from *New Delhi* age **30 yrs** reported to N.I.C.E with the symptoms of **Fever, Sore throat, Tiredness** with comorbidity like **Hypertension** got cured in **3 days** under the N.I.C.E Care of **Gopinath Narayanam**

Patient **Deepak Kumar Gupta** from *New Delhi* age **69 yrs** reported to N.I.C.E with the symptoms of **Fever, Sore throat, Tiredness** with comorbidities like **Hypertension,heart disease** got cured in **3 days** under the N.I.C.E Care of **Jitendra Ramaiya**

Patient **Indrajit Mukhraji** from *Madral* age **42 yrs** reported to N.I.C.E with the symptoms of **Fever, Dry Cough, Sore throat, Headache, Body ache/muscle ache, Tiredness** with comorbidity like **Diabetes** got cured in **3 days** under the N.I.C.E Care of **Dr Chitra Jain**

Patient **Nanak** from *New Delhi* age **44 yrs** reported to N.I.C.E with the symptoms of **Fever, Tiredness** with comorbidity like **Hypertension** got cured in **3 days** under the N.I.C.E Care of **Lomash Anand**

Patient **Rekha Gupta** from *New Delhi* age **38 yrs** reported to N.I.C.E with the symptoms of **Fever, Sore throat, Tiredness Weakness** on **07-Jun-20** with comorbidity like **Low blood pressure** got cured in **3 days** under the N.I.C.E Care of **Kanishk Amarpuri**

Patient **Somnath Todkar** from *Santacruz* age **56 yrs** reported to N.I.C.E with the symptom of extreme **Weakness** on **07-Jul-20** with comorbidities like **Diabetes & Liver Cirrhosis** got cured in **4 days** under the N.I.C.E Care of **Nishan Singh Jamwal**

Patient **Rudramallikarjun** from *Hyderabad* age **47 yrs** reported to N.I.C.E with the symptoms of **Fever, Congestion, Tiredness, breathing difficulty** with comorbidity like **Hypertension** got cured in **3 days** under the N.I.C.E Care of **Shikha Saxena**

Patient **Mandeep Singh** from *New Delhi* age **34 yrs** reported to N.I.C.E with the symptoms of **Fever, Dry Cough, Sore throat, Body ache/muscle ache, Tiredness** with comorbidities like **Hypertension and mild lungs infection** got cured in **7 days** under the N.I.C.E Care of **Biswajit Datta**

Patient **Narayansingh B.Bhandari.** from *Thane* age **50 yrs** reported to N.I.C.E with the symptom of **Weakness** on **07-Jun-20** with comorbidity like **Klebsiella Pneumoniae** got cured in **15 days** under the N.I.C.E Care of **Biswajit Datta**

Patient **Mohit Bhatia** from *New Delhi* age **37 yrs** reported to N.I.C.E with the symptom of **Sore throat** on **07-Sep-20** with comorbidity like **Ankylosing spondylitis** got cured in **3 days** under the N.I.C.E Care of **Dr Seema Arora**

Patient **Ranjeet kaur** from *New Delhi* age **60 yrs** reported to N.I.C.E with the symptoms of **Fever, Dry Cough, Headache, Body ache/muscle ache/, Tiredness Weakness** with comorbidity like **Depression** got cured in **4 days** under the N.I.C.E Care of **Rahul Bansal**

Patient **Satish Rajaji Gowda** from *Bengaluru* age **46 yrs** reported to N.I.C.E with the symptoms of **Sore throat, Body ache/muscle ache/,** on **08-Jun-20** with comorbidity like **Diabetes** got cured in **8 days** under the N.I.C.E Care of **Sushma Bengani**

Patient **Mahendra Yadav** from *Thane* age **40 yrs** reported to N.I.C.E with the symptoms of **Body ache/muscle ache, breathing difficulty** on **11-Jun-20** with comorbidity like **Hypertension** got cured in **4 days** under the N.I.C.E Care of **Kanishk Amarpuri**

Patient **Patel Amar** from *Ahmedabad* age **22 yrs** reported to N.I.C.E with the symptom of **Sore throat** on **11-Jun-20** with comorbidities like **Asthma, acidity** got cured in **3 days** under the N.I.C.E Care of **Simi Handa**

Patient **Tarun Kamra** from *Jhansi* age **57 yrs** reported to N.I.C.E with the symptom of **Sore throat** on **11-Jun-20** with comorbidities like **Hypertension, Diabetes** got cured in **7 days** under the N.I.C.E Care of **Bhupendra Singh Panwar**

Patient **Chhote Lal** from *New Delhi* age **65 yrs** reported to N.I.C.E with the symptoms of **Sore throat, Body ache/muscle ache, Congestion, Tiredness** on **11-Jun-20** with comorbidity like **Hypertension and Diabetes** got cured in **2 days** under the N.I.C.E Care of **Sayed**

Patient **Banwari** from *New Delhi* age **45 yrs** reported to N.I.C.E with the symptoms of **Sore throat, Headache,** on **12-Jun-20** with comorbidities like **Diabetes, Hypertension** got cured in **3 days** under the N.I.C.E Care of **Pratiksha Vats**

Patient **Kavita Pathak** from *New Delhi* age **27 yrs** reported to N.I.C.E with the symptom of **Body ache/muscle ache,** on **06-Dec-20** with comorbidity like **gallbladder stone,** got cured in **14 days** under the N.I.C.E Care of **Raj Kishore Kodwani**

Patient **Vishal Madaan** from *Faridabad* age **40 yrs** reported to N.I.C.E with the symptoms of **Sore throat, Body ache/muscle ache, Tiredness** with comorbidity like **Diabetes** got cured in **5 days** under the N.I.C.E Care of **Pratiksha Vats**

Patient **Naseem Ahmed** from *New Delhi* age **52 yrs** reported to N.I.C.E with the symptoms of **Tiredness, breathing difficulty** with comorbidity like **Diabetes** got cured in **4 days** under the N.I.C.E Care of **Rachna Sharma**

Patient **Anil Nerkar** from *Nallasopara* age **59 yrs** reported to N.I.C.E with the symptom of **Sore throat** with comorbidity like **Hypertension** got cured in **7 days** under the N.I.C.E Care of **Kalpana Bourai**

Patient **Sandeep Jain** from *New Delhi* age **52 yrs** reported to N.I.C.E with the symptoms of **Fever, Headache, Tiredness** with comorbidities like **Hypertension, Diabetes** got cured in **10 days** under the N.I.C.E Care of **Rameshwar Thokchom**

Patient **Praveen Kumar** from *Aurangabad* age **51 yrs** reported to N.I.C.E with the symptom of **breathing difficulty** with comorbidity like **Hypertension** got cured in **5 days** under the N.I.C.E Care of **Emmanuel Job**

Patient **Kapil Dev** from *Narela* age **38 yrs** reported to N.I.C.E with the symptoms of **Dry Cough, Sore throat, Headache, Body ache/ muscle ache, Tiredness** with comorbidities like **Hypertension, Diabetes** got cured in **6 days** under the N.I.C.E Care of **Emmanuel Job**

Patient **Braham singh** from *New Delhi* age **65 yrs** reported to N.I.C.E with the symptoms of **Fever, Sore throat, Body ache/ muscle ache** on **06-May-20** with comorbidity like **Hypertension** got cured in **11 days** under the N.I.C.E Care of **Hulash Chand Sankhla**

Patient **Naveen** from *New Delhi* age **35 yrs** reported to N.I.C.E with the symptoms of **Fever, Sore throat, Body ache/muscle ache, Tiredness** with comorbidity like **Hypertension** got cured in **3 days** under the N.I.C.E Care of **Hulash Chand Sankhla**

Patient **Sudhir Kumar** from *Dhanbad* age **37 yrs** reported to N.I.C.E with the symptoms of **Fever, Body ache/muscle ache** with comorbidities like **Thyroid, Jaundice** got cured in **4 days** under the N.I.C.E Care of **Dr Goutam Paul**

Patient **Salma Khatoon** from *Kolkata* age **58 yrs** reported to N.I.C.E with the symptoms of **Dry Cough, Body ache/muscle ache, breathing difficulty** with c comorbidity like **Hypertension** got cured in **7 days** under the N.I.C.E Care of **Avinash Popatrao Sabare**

Patient **Kamalaprasad Maurya** from *Goregaon* age **67 yrs** reported to N.I.C.E with the symptoms of **Dry Cough, Sore throat, Body ache/muscle ache, Breathing difficulty** on 10-Jan-53 with comorbidity like **Diabetes** got cured in **6 days** under the N.I.C.E Care of **Pratiksha Vats**

Patient **Dewati Thapa** from *Faridabad* age **51 yrs** reported to N.I.C.E with the symptoms of **Fever, Sore throat, Headache, Body ache/muscle ache** with comorbidity like **Thyroid** got cured in **9 days** under the N.I.C.E Care of **Hemraj Jagannath Saner**

Patient **Vikash kumar** from *Lucknow* age **36 yrs** reported to N.I.C.E with the symptom of **Tiredness** on 18-Jun-20 with comorbidity like **Depression** got cured in **2 days** under the N.I.C.E Care of **Hulash Chand Sankhla**

Patient **Vijaykumar L Valand** from *Vadodara* age **52 yrs** reported to N.I.C.E with the symptoms of **Fever, Body ache/muscle ache/, Weakness** on 07-Jun-20 with comorbidity like **Diabetes** got cured in **0 days** under the N.I.C.E Care of **Kanishk Amarpuri**

Patient **Nandkishore Darak** from *Bengaluru* age **57 yrs** reported to N.I.C.E with the symptoms of **Fever, Dry Cough** on 21-Jun-20 with comorbidity like **Diabetes** got cured in **4 days** under the N.I.C.E Care of **Seema Manikkoth**

Patient **Anil mansukhabhai patel** from *Mumbai* age **46 yrs** reported to N.I.C.E with the symptom of **Dry Cough** on 12-Jul-20 with c comorbidity like **Hypertension** got cured in **6 days** under the N.I.C.E Care of **Nishu Sandhya**

Patient **Maharani Devi** from *Agra* age **66 yrs** reported to N.I.C.E with the symptoms of **Fever, Dry Cough, Sore throat, Headache, Body ache/muscle ache, Congestion, Tiredness** on 27-Jun-20 with comorbidities like **Diabetes, Hypertension** got cured in **7 days** under the N.I.C.E Care of **Adarsha Narayan Pradhan**

Patient **Nadim Saba Prawaz** from *New Delhi* age **56 yrs** reported to N.I.C.E with the symptoms of **Fever, Dry Cough, Sore throat, Headache, Body ache/muscle ache, Congestion, Tiredness, breathing difficulty** on **16-Jun-20** with comorbidities like **Diabetes, hypertension and Asthma** got cured in **4 days** under the N.I.C.E Care of **Vinod Kumar Katheria**

Patient **Rahul Pandey** from *Dhanbad* age **29 yrs** reported to N.I.C.E with the symptoms of **Fever, Tiredness Weakness** on **08-Jul-20** with comorbidity like **Epilepsy** got cured in **3 days** under the N.I.C.E Care of **Pragya Jha**

Patient **Omprakash agarwal** from *Kalyan* age **44 yrs** reported to N.I.C.E with the suspected symptoms influenza of on **01-Jul-20** with comorbidity like **Hypertension** got cured in **4 days** under the N.I.C.E Care of **Biswajit Datta**

Patient **Kamlakar Power** from *Kalyan* age **56 yrs** reported to N.I.C.E with the symptoms of **Body ache/muscle ache/, Tiredness breathing difficulty, Weakness** on **03-Jul-20** with comorbidity like **Diabetes** got cured in **5 days** under the N.I.C.E Care of **Biswajit Datta**

Patient **Vasundhara Vasantrao Jadhav** from *Daund* age **78 yrs** reported to N.I.C.E with the symptoms of **Fever, Dry Cough, Sore throat, Headache, Body ache/muscle ache/, Congestion, Tiredness Weakness** on **07-Jul-20** with comorbidities like **Hypertension,Piles** got cured in **7 days** under the N.I.C.E Care of **Suresh Kumar Yadav**

Patient **Nishi Prashad** from *Hyderabad* age **48 yrs** reported to N.I.C.E with the symptoms of **Fever, Sore throat, Body ache/ muscle ache, Tiredness, Weakness** on **04-Jul-20** with comorbidity like **borderline diabetes** got cured in **4 days** under the N.I.C.E Care of **Dr. Vishwajeet Khaiwal**

Patient **V.Ellari** from *Hyderabad* age **50 yrs** reported to N.I.C.E with the symptom of **Dry Cough** on **07-Jun-20** with comorbidity like **Hypertension** got cured in **4 days** under the N.I.C.E Care of **Bhagwan Dass**

Patient **Ramadhar Patel** from *Rewa* age **75 yrs** reported to N.I.C.E with the symptoms of **Fever, Headache, Body ache/muscle ache, Tiredness** on **27-Jun-20** with comorbidity like **Hypertension** got cured in **7 days** under the N.I.C.E Care of **Ayan haldar**

Patient **Dilip Kumar Paul** from *Siliguri* age **78 yrs** reported to N.I.C.E with the symptoms of **Fever, Dry Cough, Sore throat, Headache, Body ache/muscle ache/, Tiredness Weakness** on **09-Jul-20** with comorbidities like **Hypertension, heart disease, diabetes, prostate** got cured in **4 days** under the N.I.C.E Care of **Dr. Madan Lal**

Patient **Swapan Dey** from *Kolkata* age **71 yrs** reported to N.I.C.E with the symptoms of **Fever, Dry Cough, Body ache/muscle ache/, Weakness** on **09-Jul-20** with comorbidity like **Hypertension** got cured in **5 days** under the N.I.C.E Care of **Dr. Madan Lal**

Patient **Bhupinder Singh** from *Ludhiana* age **48 yrs** reported to N.I.C.E with the symptom of **Sore throat** on **26-Jun-20** with comorbidity like **Hypertension** got cured in **4 days** under the N.I.C.E Care of **Chitra jain**

Patient **Jayesh Kadare** from *Navi Mumbai* age **36 yrs** reported to N.I.C.E with the symptoms of **Fever, Dry Cough, Headache, Body ache/muscle ache/, Tiredness Weakness** on **07-Jul-20** with comorbidity like **Psoriasis** got cured in **6 days** under the N.I.C.E Care of **Sayed Shah**

Patient **Rituraj Mauarya** from *Surat* age **27 yrs** reported to N.I.C.E with the symptoms of **Congestion, breathing difficulty** on **09-Jul-20** with comorbidity like **Asthma** got cured in **4 days** under the N.I.C.E Care of **Dr Seema Arora**

Patient **Anand Datta** from *New Delhi* age **72 yrs** reported to N.I.C.E with the symptom of **Congestion** on **03-Jul-20** with comorbidities like **Swollen Liver and Hypertension** got cured in **7 days** under the N.I.C.E Care of **Brijmohan Yadav**

Patient **Kauser Begum** from *Hyderabad* age **40 yrs** reported to N.I.C.E with the symptoms of **Fever, Congestion, Tiredness, breathing difficulty** on 30-Jun-20 with comorbidities like **Diabetes, Thyroid,** got cured in **6 days** under the N.I.C.E Care of **Goma Ram**

Patient **Kolhe Sunil Suryabhan** from *Pune* age 51 yrs reported to N.I.C.E with the symptoms of **Dry Cough, Sore throat, Headache, Body ache/muscle ache/** on 05-Jul-20 with comorbidity like **Hypertension** got cured in **4 days** under the N.I.C.E Care of **Ashish**

Patient **Chetna** from *Mumbai* age **43 yrs** reported to N.I.C.E with the symptoms of **Fever, Sore throat, Congestion, breathing difficulty** on 07-Jan-20 got cured in **7 days** under the N.I.C.E Care of **Suresh Kumar Yadav**

Patient **Deepak Dodeja** from *ulhasnagar1.thane..mumbai* age 37 yrs reported to N.I.C.E with the symptoms of **Fever, Weakness** on 07-Jul-20 with comorbidity like **Hypertension** got cured in **7 days** under the N.I.C.E Care of **Suresh Kumar Yadav**

Patient **Kantaben Mudusudan** from *Ahmedabad* age **72 yrs** reported to N.I.C.E with the symptoms of **Fever, Dry Cough, Headache, Body ache/muscle ache/, Congestion, Tiredness Weakness** on 04-Jul-20 with comorbidity like **Diabetes,** got cured in **6 days** under the N.I.C.E Care of **Kimti Lal**

Patient **Mhash jain** from *New Delhi* age 58 yrs reported to N.I.C.E with the symptoms of **Fever, Headache, Body ache/muscle ache, Tiredness** on 18-Jun-20 with comorbidity like **Thyroid** got cured in **4 days** under the N.I.C.E Care of **Kimti Lal**

Patient **Deepa** from *New Delhi* age **58 yrs** reported to N.I.C.E with the symptoms of **Fever, Headache, Body ache/muscle ache, Tiredness** on 18-Jun-20 with comorbidity like **Thyroid** got cured in **7 days** under the N.I.C.E Care of **Kimti Lal**

Patient **Gyanchand** from *Chennai* age 57 yrs reported to N.I.C.E with the symptoms of **Fever, Dry Cough, Congestion, Tiredness breathing difficulty** on 12-Jul-20 with comorbidities like **Diabetes** and heart diseae got cured in **7 days** under the N.I.C.E Care of **Shiv Dular**

Patient **Banjul Barthakur** from *Jorhat* age **57 yrs** reported to N.I.C.E with the symptoms of **Fever, Dry Cough, Sore throat, Body ache/muscle ache/, Tiredness Weakness** on 11-Jul-20 with comorbidities like **Hypertension,mild blockage in arteries** got cured in **3 days** under the N.I.C.E Care of **Dr Seema Arora**

Patient **V. Ananthanarayanan** from *Chennai* age **59 yrs** reported to N.I.C.E with the symptoms of **Fever, Body ache/muscle ache/, Tiredness** on **08-Jul-20** with comorbidity like **Diabetes** got cured in **5 days** under the N.I.C.E Care of **Goma Ram**

Patient **Mr. A A Samarth** from *Ambarnath* age **48 yrs** reported to N.I.C.E with the symptoms of **Body ache/muscle ache, Tiredness** on **30-Jun-20** with comorbidities like **Hypertension, Diabetes** got cured in **7 days** under the N.I.C.E Care of **Ekta agarwal**

Patient **Siyaram Singh** from *Paliganj* age **59 yrs** reported to N.I.C.E with the symptoms of **Fever, Headache, Weakness** on 10-Jul-20 with comorbidity like **Diabetes** got cured in **6 days** under the N.I.C.E Care of **Nishan Singh Jamwal**

Patient **Nandkumar Ramasing** from *Bhayender west* age **35 yrs** reported to N.I.C.E with the symptom of **Fever** on 23-Jun-20 with comorbidity like **Hypertension** got cured in **4 days** under the N.I.C.E Care of **Kavitha N Jain**

Patient **Mahira Afreen** from *Melbourne* age **23 yrs** reported to N.I.C.E with the symptoms of **Fever, Dry Cough, Sore throat, Headache, Body ache/muscle ache** on **17-Sep-97** with comorbidity like **Sinusitis** got cured in **6 days** under the N.I.C.E Care of **Kavitha N Jain**

Patient **Nandini Thorat** from *Aurangabad* age **3 yrs** reported to N.I.C.E with the symptoms of **Fever, Tiredness Weakness** on 10-Jul-20 got cured in **7 days** under the N.I.C.E Care of **Kapil Dev Sharma**

Patient **Manju Latha** from *Bengaluru* age **36 yrs** reported to N.I.C.E with the symptom of **Dry Cough** on **07-Jul-20** with comorbidity like **Hypothyriod** got cured in **4 days** under the N.I.C.E Care of **Bhagwan Dass**

Patient **Shreekanya Kodate** from *Pune* age **25 yrs** reported to N.I.C.E with the symptoms of **Fever, Sore throat, Headache** on **10-Jul-20** with comorbidities like **allergy** got cured in **7 days** under the N.I.C.E Care of **Bimal Pal**

Patient **Shankar Agarwal** from **Kol** age **29 yrs** reported to N.I.C.E with **Corona positive reports** on **29-Jun-20** got cured in **6 days** under the N.I.C.E Care of **Sayed Shah**

Patient **Ashok** from **Uran** age **30 yrs** reported to N.I.C.E with the symptoms of **Fever, Dry Cough, Tiredness, Weakness** on **11-Jul-20** got cured in **4 days** under the N.I.C.E Care of **Dr. Kishan Pareek**

Patient **Neel shah** from **Valsad** age **19 yrs** reported to N.I.C.E with the symptoms of **Fever, Headache** on **11-Jul-20** got cured in **3 days** under the N.I.C.E Care of **Sayed Shah**

Patient **Devaki B. Rewadkar** from **Mumbai** age **61 yrs** reported to N.I.C.E with the symptoms of **Fever, Headache, Body ache/muscle ache, Tiredness** on **30-Jun-20** got cured in **7 days** under the N.I.C.E Care of **Arun Kumar**

Patient **Prasant Kumar** from **Mumbai** age **26 yrs** reported to N.I.C.E with the symptoms of **Fever, Headache, Body ache/muscle ache, Tiredness** on **11-Jul-20** got cured in **4 days** under the N.I.C.E Care of **Dr. Kishan Pareek**

Patient **Saurabh** from **Lalitpur** age **35 yrs** reported to N.I.C.E with the symptoms of **Fever, Sore throat, Body ache/muscle ache, Weakness** on **11-Jul-20** got cured in **3 days** under the N.I.C.E Care of **Dr. Kishan Pareek**

Patient **Aakash kamble** from **Navi Mumbai** age **35 yrs** reported to N.I.C.E with the symptoms of **Fever, Headache, Body ache/muscle** ache, Tiredness, Weakness on 11-Jul-20 got cured in 4 days under the N.I.C.E Care of **Dr. Kishan Pareek**

Patient **Jagruti Singh** from **Kalyan West**, age **26 yrs** reported to N.I.C.E with the symptoms of **Fever, Dry Cough, Headache, Congestion, Tiredness** on 08-Jul-20 got cured in 3 days under the N.I.C.E Care of **Dr. Kishan Pareek**

Patient **Syed Abdul Gaffar** from **Hyderabad** age **38 yrs** reported to N.I.C.E with the symptoms of **Fever, Congestion** on 13-Jul-20 got cured in **7 days** under the N.I.C.E Care of **Bhagwan Dass**

Patient **Kishore Kataria** from **Bengaluru** age **48 yrs** reported to N.I.C.E with the symptoms of **Fever, Dry Cough, Sore throat, Headache, Body ache/muscle ache, Tiredness, Weakness** on 04-Jul-20 got cured in **6 days** under the N.I.C.E Care of **Rajwinder Kaur**

Patient **Rohan** from **Mysore** age **2 yrs** reported to N.I.C.E with the symptoms of **Fever** on 11-Jul-20 got cured in **5 days** under the N.I.C.E Care of **Filda Don**

Patient **ansari arif** from **Bhiwandi** age **42 yrs** reported to N.I.C.E with the symptoms of **Fever, Dry Cough, Body ache/muscle ache, Tiredness, Breathing difficulty** on 02-Jul-20 got cured in **6 days** under the N.I.C.E Care of **Rahul Bansal**

Patient **rinki shaw de** from **Kolkata** age **32 yrs** reported to N.I.C.E with the symptoms of **Dry Cough, Headache, Weakness** on 10-Jul-20 got cured in **3 days.**

Patient **sachinder singh** from **Patna** age **31 yrs** reported to N.I.C.E with the symptoms of **Dry Cough, Sore throat, Breathing difficulty** on 10-Jul-20 got cured in **6 days** under the N.I.C.E Care of **Rahul Bansal**

Patient **Samir** from **Mandsaur** age **32 yrs** reported to N.I.C.E with the symptoms of **Fever, Body ache/muscle ache, Tiredness, Weakness** on **09-Jul-20** got cured in **6 days** under the N.I.C.E Care of **Biswajit Datta**

Patient **Santosh Narayan Ugile** from **Hydrabad** age **33 yrs** reported to N.I.C.E with the symptoms of **Body ache/muscle ache** on 07-Jul-20 got cured in **6 days** under the N.I.C.E Care of **Biswajit Datta**

Patient **Nandini Yashodeep** from **Aurangabad** age **2 yrs** reported to N.I.C.E with the symptom of **Fever** on **10-Jul-20** got cured in **6 days** under the N.I.C.E Care of **Rahul Bansal**

Patient **Nikhi Goyal** from **Kolkata** age **35 yrs** reported to N.I.C.E with the symptoms of **Fever, Dry Cough, Body ache/muscle ache, Tiredness, Weakness** on 06-Jul-20 got cured in **5 days** under the N.I.C.E Care of **Rahul Bansal**

Patient **Suphiyan** from **Pune** age **34 yrs** reported to N.I.C.E with the symptoms of **Fever, Body ache/muscle ache, Weakness** on 06-Jul-20 got cured in **3 days** under the N.I.C.E Care of **Rahul Bansal**

Patient **Prashant Kumbhar** from **Pune** age **34 yrs** reported to N.I.C.E with the symptoms of **Fever, Body ache/muscle ache, Weakness** on 06-Jul-20 got cured in **3 days** under the N.I.C.E Care of **Rahul Bansal**

Patient **Shubham Thakur** from **Sirali** age **26 yrs** reported to N.I.C.E with the symptom of **Tiredness** on **11-Jul-20** got cured in **6 days** under the N.I.C.E Care of **Suresh Kumar Yadav**

Patient **Rohit Kad** from **Pune** age **29 yrs** reported to N.I.C.E with the symptoms of **Dry Cough, Sore throat** on 11-Jul-20 got cured in **4 days** under the N.I.C.E Care of **Suresh Kumar Yadav**

Patient **Sudhir Thorat** from **Kalyan** age **52 yrs** reported to N.I.C.E with the symptoms of **Dry Cough, Congestion, Tiredness, Breathing difficulty, Weakness** on 10-Jul-20 got cured in **4 days** under the N.I.C.E Care of **Ashish**

Patient **Sunny Manchanda** from **Nashik** age **35 yrs** reported to N.I.C.E with the symptoms of **Tiredness, Breathing difficulty** on 11-Jul-20 got cured in **7 days** under the N.I.C.E Care of **Ashish**

Patient **Shiv prasad swami** from **Pune** age **26 yrs** reported to N.I.C.E with the symptoms of **Dry Cough, Sore throat, Headache, Body ache/muscle ache** on **12-Jul-20** got cured in **3 days** under the N.I.C.E Care of **Ashish**

Patient **Rajkumar Swami** from **Pune** age **28 yrs** reported to N.I.C.E with the symptoms of **Sore throat, Headache, Body ache/muscle ache, Congestion, Tiredness** on **13-Jul-20** got cured in **4 days** under the N.I.C.E Care of **Ashish**

Patient **Hardik Mudi** from **East Singhbum** age **4 yrs** reported to N.I.C.E with the symptoms of **Fever, Headache** on **14-Jul-20** got cured in **6 days** under the N.I.C.E Care of **Ashish**

Patient **A.Akshara reddy** from **Secunderabad** age **18 yrs** reported to N.I.C.E with the symptom of **Sore throat** on **10-Jul-20** got cured in **7 days** under the N.I.C.E Care of **Gopinath Narayanam**

Patient **Arun Kumar** from **New delhi** age **27 yrs** reported to N.I.C.E with the symptoms of **Sore throat, Headache, Congestion, Breathing difficulty, Weakness** on **02-Jul-20** got cured in **5 days** under the N.I.C.E Care of **Gopinath Narayanam**

Patient **Ajit Kumar** from **Varanasi** age **54 yrs** reported to N.I.C.E with the symptoms of **Fever, Dry Cough, Sore throat, Headache, Body ache/muscle ache, Tiredness** on **11-Jul-20** got cured in **3 days** under the N.I.C.E Care of **Kamlakshi Shahdeo**

Patient **Hamsa** from **Bengaluru** age **45 yrs** reported to N.I.C.E with the symptoms of **Fever, Dry Cough, Sore throat, Headache, Body ache/muscle ache, Congestion, Tiredness, Breathing difficulty, Weakness** on **12-Jul-20** got cured in **5 days** under the N.I.C.E Care of **Kamlakshi Shahdeo**

Patient **Sanjana Anand** from **Chennai** age **26 yrs** reported to N.I.C.E with the symptoms of **Fever, Sore throat, Body ache/muscle ache, Tiredness, Breathing difficulty, Weakness** on **06-Jul-20** got cured in **6 days** under the N.I.C.E Care of **Gopinath Narayanam**

Patient **D. Janaki Raghava** from **Hyderabad** age **28 yrs** reported to N.I.C.E with the symptoms of **Headache, Weakness** on **26-Jun-20** got cured in **7 days** under the N.I.C.E Care of **Gopinath Narayanam**

Patient **Akash Mali** from **Pune** age **25 yrs** reported to N.I.C.E with the symptoms of **Fever, Sore throat, Headache, Congestion, Tiredness, Weakness** on **12-Jul-20** got cured in **3 days** under the N.I.C.E Care of **Kamlakshi Shahdeo**

Patient **Alok Sharma** from **Kolkata** age **30 yrs** reported to N.I.C.E with the symptoms of **Dry Cough, Sore throat, Tiredness** on **01-Jul-20** got cured in **5 days** under the N.I.C.E Care of **Jitendra Ramaiya**

Patient **Swapnil Arun bire** from **Pune** age **22 yrs** reported to N.I.C.E with the symptoms of **Dry Cough, Headache, Body ache/ muscle ache, Tiredness, c** on **31-Jul-20** got cured in **7 days** under the N.I.C.E Care of **Jitendra Ramaiya**

Patient **Jitendra Bharatwa** from **Kalyan** age **54 yrs** reported to N.I.C.E with the symptoms of **Fever, Headache, Body ache/muscle ache, Weakness** on **13-Jul-20** got cured in **3 days** under the N.I.C.E Care of **B.Narendran**

Patient **Reetu** from **Barabanki** age **35 yrs** reported to N.I.C.E with the symptoms of **Fever, Headache, Body ache/muscle ache, Tiredness, Weakness** on **11-Jul-20** got cured in **3 days** under the N.I.C.E Care of **Sounak Das**

Patient **Rohith** from **Hyderabad** age **20 yrs** reported to N.I.C.E with the symptoms of **Fever, Dry Cough, Sore throat, Headache, Body ache/muscle ache, Tiredness, Breathing difficulty, Weakness** on **11-Jul-20** got cured in **3 days** under the N.I.C.E Care of **Alisha Massey**

Patient **Mayur Jadhav** from **Surat** age **23 yrs** reported to N.I.C.E with the symptoms of **Sore throat, Congestion, Weakness** on **10-Jul-20** got cured in **4 days** under the N.I.C.E Care of **Brijmohan Yadav**

Patient **Dr Harshali Pawar** from **Kalyan** age **29 yrs** reported to N.I.C.E with the symptom of **Breathing difficulty** on **24-Jun-20** got cured in **4 days** under the N.I.C.E Care of **Rachna Sharma**

Patient **Sneha Singh** from **Kolkata** age **34 yrs** reported to N.I.C.E with the symptoms of **Dry Cough, Sore throat, Headache, Body ache/muscle ache, Congestion, Tiredness, Breathing difficulty** on **24-Jun-20** got cured in **3 days** under the N.I.C.E Care of **Rachna Sharma**

Patient **Sanjay Arora** from **Noida** age **45 yrs** reported to N.I.C.E with the symptoms of **Fever, Headache, Body ache/muscle ache** on **24-Jun-20** got cured in **6 days** under the N.I.C.E Care of **Jitendra Ramaiya**

Patient **Navnath Mazire** from **Pune** age **37 yrs** reported to N.I.C.E with the symptom of **Dry Cough** on **24-Jun-20** got cured in **7 days** under the N.I.C.E Care of **Kalpana Bourai**

Patient **Tejveer** from **New Delhi** age **30 yrs** reported to N.I.C.E with the symptoms of **Sore throat, Body ache/muscle ache, Tiredness, Breathing difficulty** on **22-Jun-20** got cured in **4 days** under the N.I.C.E Care of **Kalpana Bourai**

Patient **Ashok Rambhau Nikalje** from **Pune Pimpri Chinchwad** age **54 yrs** reported to N.I.C.E with the symptoms of **Fever, Dry Cough, Body ache/muscle ache** on **24-Jun-20** got cured in **7 days** under the N.I.C.E Care of **Pradeep Chauhan**

Patient **Satish Rathod** from **Korpana** age **38 yrs** reported to N.I.C.E with the symptoms of **Body ache/muscle ache, Tiredness, c** on **21-Jun-20** got cured in **4 days** under the N.I.C.E Care of **Pratiksha Vats**

Patient **Vinod Taneja** from **Faridabad** age **44 yrs** reported to N.I.C.E with the symptom of **Fever** on **20-Jun-20** got cured in **6 days** under the N.I.C.E Care of **Sounak Das**

Patient **Mohammad Zeeshan** from **Allahabad** age **22 yrs** reported to N.I.C.E with the symptoms of **Fever, Dry Cough, Headache,**

Body ache/muscle ache, Congestion, Tiredness on 21-Jun-20 got cured in **6 days** under the N.I.C.E Care of **Simi Handa**

Patient **Chandra Rekha Gupta** from **Kanpur** age **55 yrs** reported to N.I.C.E with the symptoms of **Fever, Tiredness** on 26-Jun-20 got cured in **6 days** under the N.I.C.E Care of **Hemraj Jagannath Saner**

Patient **Nitin sharma** from **Agra** age **42 yrs** reported to N.I.C.E with the symptoms of **Sore throat, Body ache/muscle ache,** on 26-Jun-20 got cured in **5 days** under the N.I.C.E Care of **Hemraj Jagannath Saner**

Patient **Gora Chowdhury** from **Kolkata** age **56 yrs** reported to N.I.C.E with the symptoms of **Fever, Tiredness** on 26-Jun-20 got cured in **3 days** under the N.I.C.E Care of **Suresh Kumar Yadav**

Patient **Pavan jain Kala** from **Hyderabad** age **56 yrs** reported to N.I.C.E with the symptoms of **Fever, Dry Cough, Headache** on 26-Jun-20 got cured in **7 days** under the N.I.C.E Care of **Gopinath Narayanam**

Patient **Jawaharlal Prajapati** from **Mumbai** age **49 yrs** reported to N.I.C.E with the symptoms of **Dry Cough, Headache, Tiredness** on 23-Jun-20 got cured in **6 days**

Patient **Atul Goswami** from **Faridabad** age **24 yrs** reported to N.I.C.E with the symptoms of **Dry Cough, Sore throat, Headache, Body ache/muscle ache, Tiredness** on 23-Jun-20 got cured in **4 days**

Patient **Krunal Vivek karambe** from **Panvel** age **20 yrs** reported to N.I.C.E with the symptoms of **Fever, Dry Cough, Headache** on 23-Jun-20 got cured in **3 days** under the N.I.C.E Care of **Samir Das**

Patient **Tushar Vashishth** from **Faridabad** age **33 yrs** reported to N.I.C.E with the symptoms of **Sore throat, Body ache/muscle ache, Tiredness** on 23-Jun-20 got cured in **5 days**

Patient **Shubham Mishra** from **New Delhi** age **24 yrs** reported to N.I.C.E with the symptoms of **Fever, Tiredness** on **22-Jun-20** got cured in **3 days** under the N.I.C.E Care of **Goma Ram**

Patient **Manish Sirture** from **Indore** age **35 yrs** reported to N.I.C.E with the symptoms of **Congestion, Tiredness, c** on **23-Jun-20** got cured in **7 days**

Patient **Ishaan Tyagi** from **Ghaziabad** age **16 yrs** reported to N.I.C.E with the symptoms of **Headache** on **23-Jun-20** got cured in **7 days**

Patient **Ashwani** from **Allahabad** age **26 yrs** reported to N.I.C.E with the symptoms of **Breathing difficulty** on **23-Jun-20** got cured in **5 days**

Patient **Sandeep Gulia** from **Faridabad** age **37 yrs** reported to N.I.C.E with the symptoms of **Fever, Body ache/muscle ache, Tiredness** on **23-Jun-20** got cured in **4 days** under the N.I.C.E Care of **Girish Banvi**

Patient **Surjeet Singh** from **Kaimganj** age **1950 yrs** reported to N.I.C.E with the symptoms of **Dry Cough, Headache** on **23-Jun-20** got cured in **7 days.**

Patient **Vinod** from **New Delhi** age **34 yrs** reported to N.I.C.E with the symptoms of **Fever, Headache, Body ache/muscle ache, Congestion, Tiredness** on **23-Jun-20** got cured in **4 days** under the N.I.C.E Care of **Prabhjot Kaur**

Patient **Ramesh Kumar** from **Gurugram** age **48 yrs** reported to N.I.C.E with the symptoms of **Fever, Body ache/muscle ache** on **23-Jun-20** got cured in **7 days** under the N.I.C.E Care of **Sanjay Gupta**

Patient **Jai Prakash Yadav** from **Ghaziabad** age **40 yrs** reported to N.I.C.E with the symptoms of **Dry Cough, Headache, Tiredness** on **23-Jun-20** got cured in **4 days.**

Patient **Balasaheb Survase** from **Aurangabad** age **55 yrs** reported to N.I.C.E with the symptom of **Dry Cough** on **23-Jun-20** got cured in **6 days**

Patient **Sanchit Patil** from **Pune** age **26 yrs** reported to N.I.C.E with the symptoms of **Fever, Headache, Body ache/muscle ache** on **23-Jun-20** got cured in **4 days** under the N.I.C.E Care of **Rajendra Patil**

Patient **Mangesh Devre** from **Kalyan** age **52 yrs** reported to N.I.C.E with the symptom of **Dry Cough** on **24-Jun-20** got cured in **4 days**

Patient **Mohd Iqbal** from **Jodhpur** age **65 yrs** reported to N.I.C.E with the symptoms of **Dry Cough, Breathing difficulty** on **24-Jun-20** got cured in **5 days**

Patient **Syed Ali** from **Hyderabad** age **39 yrs** reported to N.I.C.E with the symptoms of **Fever, Dry Cough, Sore throat, Body ache/muscle ache, Tiredness** on **28-Jun-20** got cured in **4 days** under the N.I.C.E Care of **Bhagwan Dass**

Patient **Sanoop Singh Negi** from **New Delhi** age **28 yrs** reported to N.I.C.E with the symptom of **Dry Cough** on **26-Jun-20** got cured in **6 days** under the N.I.C.E Care of **Siddharth Jain**

Patient **Mohd Rahath** from **Hyderabad** age **28 yrs** reported to N.I.C.E with the symptoms of **Fever, Tiredness** on **28-Jun-20** got cured in **6 days** under the N.I.C.E Care of **Simi Handa**

Patient **Dattaram S Apankar** from **Mumbai** age **68 yrs** reported to N.I.C.E with the symptoms of **Fever, Body ache/muscle ache, Breathing difficulty** on **28-Jun-20** got cured in **7 days** under the N.I.C.E Care of **Ritu Singh**

Patient **Shahreyar Shareef** from **Hyderabad** age **30 yrs** reported to N.I.C.E with the symptoms of **Fever, Dry Cough, Sore throat, Body ache/muscle ache, Tiredness** on **28-Jun-20** got cured in **4 days** .

Patient **Ahmed** from **Hyderabad** age **23 yrs** reported to N.I.C.E with the symptoms of **Fever, Dry Cough, Body ache/muscle ache** on **29-Jun-20** got cured in **4 days** under the N.I.C.E Care of **Rupesh Kumar**

Patient **Pawan Kumar** from **New Delhi** age **32 yrs** reported to N.I.C.E with the symptoms of **Fever, Dry Cough, Sore throat** on **26-Jun-20** got cured in **4 days** under the N.I.C.E Care of **Madhuri Anand Kinikar**

Patient **Rajesh jain** from *Howrah* age **48 yrs** reported to N.I.C.E with the symptoms of **Fever, Dry Cough, Headache** on **11-Jul-20** with comorbidities like **Hypertension,Diabetes** got cured in **7 days** under the N.I.C.E Care of **Sayed Shah**

Patient **Rahul Raj** from *Patna* age **17 yrs** reported to N.I.C.E with the symptoms of **Fever, Headache** on **18-Jun-20** with comorbidity like **chronic headache** got cured in **5 days** under the N.I.C.E Care of **Sheetal kanwar**

Patient **Gopal** from *Vadodara* age **70 yrs** reported to N.I.C.E with the symptoms of **Fever, Headache, Body ache/muscle ache, Tiredness** on **11-Jul-20** with comorbidities like **Hypertension,diabetes,heart diseases,kidney stones** got cured in **5 days** under the N.I.C.E Care of **Dr. Kishan Pareek**

Patient **usha tirthkar** from *Solapur* age **54 yrs** reported to N.I.C.E with the symptom of **Dry Cough** on **11-Jul-20** with comorbidity like **Hypertension** got cured in **6 days** under the N.I.C.E Care of **Samir Das**

Patient **Kishor Jagtap** from *Pune* age **45 yrs** reported to N.I.C.E with the symptoms of **Fever, Headache, Body ache/muscle ache, Tiredness, Weakness** on **11-Jul-20** with comorbidity like **Sinusitis** got cured in **7 days** under the N.I.C.E Care of **Bhagwan Dass**

Patient **Margi Panchal** from *Ahmedabad* age **54 yrs** reported to N.I.C.E with the symptoms of **Fever, Sore throat, Headache, Body ache/muscle ache, Tiredness, Breathing difficulty** on **19-Jun-20** with comorbidities like **Hypertension, thyroid** got cured in **3 days** under the N.I.C.E Care of **Ranjan Ghosh**

Patient **Lalit Kumar Singvi** from *Kolkata* age **53 yrs** reported to N.I.C.E with the symptoms of **Fever, Dry Cough, Sore throat** on **21-Jun-20** with comorbidities like **Hypertension,heart disease** got cured in **4 days** under the N.I.C.E Care of **Kapil Dev Sharma**

Patient **Sonam palmu Denzongpa** from *Kolkata* age **31 yrs** reported to N.I.C.E with the symptom of **Sore throat** on 10-Jul-20 with comorbidity like **Low blood pressure** got cured in **7 days** under the N.I.C.E Care of **Biswajit Datta**

Patient **Praveen Goel** from *Delhi* age **53 yrs** reported to N.I.C.E with the symptoms of **Tiredness, Weakness** on **06-Jul-20** with comorbidity like **Hypertension** got cured in **7** days under the N.I.C.E Care of **Biswajit Datta**

Patient **RK** from *Varanasi* age **51 yrs** reported to N.I.C.E with the symptoms of **Fever, Dry Cough, Body ache/muscle ache** on **01-Jul-20** with comorbidities like **Kidney disease, Diabetes, Hypertension** got cured in **4 days** under the N.I.C.E Care of **Rahul Bansal**

Patient **Shalu** from *New Delhi* age **31 yrs** reported to N.I.C.E with the symptoms of **Fever, Sore throat, Congestion, Breathing difficulty, Weakness** on **06-Jul-20** with comorbidy like **Thyroid** got cured in **3 days** under the N.I.C.E Care of **Gopinath Narayanam**

Patient **Pratikisha Jawalkar** from *Bhiwandi* age **43 yrs** reported to N.I.C.E with the symptoms of **Fever, Congestion, Weakness** on 06-Jul-20 with comorbidity like **Anemia** got cured in **3 days** under the N.I.C.E Care of **Dr ABMK Vara Prasad**

Patient **Akshay** from *Kalyan* age **25 yrs** reported to N.I.C.E with the symptoms of **Fever, Sore throat, Body ache/muscle ache, Tiredness, Breathing difficulty, Weakness** on **04-Jul-20** with comorbidity like **Hypertension** got cured in **6 days** under the N.I.C.E Care of **Nirmala Pandey**

Patient **Pinkal H Shah** from *Mumbai* age **37 yrs** reported to N.I.C.E with the symptoms of **Dry Cough, Sore throat, Tiredness, Breathing difficulty** on **24-Jun-20** with comorbidities like **Hypertension, thyroid** got cured in **7 days** under the N.I.C.E Care of **Rachna Sharma**

Patient **Anis fatima** from *Hyderabad* age **44 yrs** reported to N.I.C.E with the symptoms of **Fever, Headache, Body ache/muscle ache, Tiredness** on **24-Jun-20** with comorbidities like **Diabetes and hypothyroidism** got cured in **7 days** under the N.I.C.E Care of **Atul Jain**

Patient **Shalini rasal** from *Borivali West* age **78 yrs** reported to N.I.C.E with the symptoms of **Fever, Body ache/muscle ache, Tiredness, Breathing difficulty** on **24-Jun-20** with comorbidity like **Diabetes** got cured in **6 days** under the N.I.C.E Care of **Nirmala Pandey**

Patient **Sanjeev kapur** from *New Delhi* age **54 yrs** reported to N.I.C.E with the symptoms of **Fever, Dry Cough, Sore throat, Headache, Body ache/muscle ache** on 24-Jun-20 with comorbidity like **Hypertension** got cured in **4 days** under the N.I.C.E Care of **Pradeep chauhan**

Patient **Prabhat Kumar** from *Uttam Nagar* age **24 yrs** reported to N.I.C.E with the symptoms of **Dry Cough, Sore throat** on 24-Jun-20 with comorbidity like **Anxiety** got cured in **6 days** under the N.I.C.E Care of **Amit Aneja**

Patient **Rama Sharma** from *New Delhi* age **33 yrs** reported to N.I.C.E with the symptoms of **Fever, Dry Cough, Sore throat, Body ache/muscle ache, Tiredness, Breathing difficulty** on 19-Jun-20 with comorbidity like **Low Blood Pressure** got cured in **3 days** under the N.I.C.E Care of **Chitra jain**

Patient **Samir Verma** from *Gopiganj* age **48 yrs** reported to N.I.C.E with the symptoms of **Dry Cough, Sore throat, Headache, Congestion, Tiredness, Breathing difficulty** on **26-Jun-20** with comorbidity like **Diabetes** got cured in **4 days** under the N.I.C.E Care of **Hemraj Jagannath Saner**

Patient **Mohammed Mohsin** from *Hyderabad* age **46 yrs** reported to N.I.C.E with the symptoms of **Fever, Headache, Body ache/ muscle ache** on **26-Jun-20** with comorbidity like **Diabetes** got cured in **4 days** under the N.I.C.E Care of **Simi Handa**

Patient **Reetu Jain** from *New Delhi* age **41 yrs** reported to N.I.C.E with the symptoms of **Sore throat, Body ache/muscle ache** on **26-Jun-20** with comorbidity like **Diabetes** got cured in **6 days** under the N.I.C.E Care of **Hemraj Jagannath Saner**

Patient **Rinku Barua** from *Faridabad* age **44 yrs** reported to N.I.C.E with the symptom of **Fever** on **26-Jun-20** with comorbidities like **Low Blood Pressure and thyroid** got cured in **6 days** under the N.I.C.E Care of **Gopinath Narayanam**

Patient **Tilak Chandra Nath** from *New Delhi* age **61 yrs** reported to N.I.C.E with the symptoms of **Body ache/muscle ache, Congestion, Tiredness, Breathing difficulty** on **26-Jun-20** with comorbidity like **Diabetes** got cured in **4 days** under the N.I.C.E Care of **Ajit Kumar Burnwal**

Patient **B Gupta** from *Kolkata* age **51 yrs** reported to N.I.C.E with the symptoms of **Fever, Body ache/muscle ache, Congestion, Tiredness** on **23-Jun-20** with comorbidity like **Diabetes** got cured in **6 days** under the N.I.C.E Care of **Samir Das**

Patient **Idrish Mansuri** from *Ahmedabad* age **49 yrs** reported to N.I.C.E with the symptoms of **Fever, Tiredness** on **23-Jun-20** with comorbidity like **Diabetes** got cured in **6 days** under the N.I.C.E Care of **Sanjay Gupta**

Patient **Dinesh** from *Hyderabad* age **52 yrs** reported to N.I.C.E with the symptoms of **Fever, Headache** on **23-Jun-20** with comorbidities like **Hypertension, Hyper Acidity** got cured in **6 days** under the N.I.C.E Care of **Sanjay Gupta**

Patient **Pushplata Sharma** from *New Delhi* age **80 yrs** reported to N.I.C.E with the symptoms of **Fever, Dry Cough** on **23-Jun-20** with comorbidities like **Hypertension, heart** got cured in **6 days** under the N.I.C.E Care of **Avinash Popatrao Sabare**

Patient **Rajesh Burad** from *Malkapur* age **60 yrs** reported to N.I.C.E with the symptoms of **Fever, Dry Cough, Sore throat, Congestion, Tiredness** on **16-Jun-20** with comorbidity like **Hypertension** got cured in **3 days** under the N.I.C.E Care of **Arvind Kumar Plaha**

Patient **Sanjeev Kumar** from *New Delhi* age **48 yrs** reported to N.I.C.E with the symptoms of **Body ache/muscle ache, Tiredness** on **24-Jun-20** with comorbidities like **Hypertension, diabetes , anxiety , thyroid** got cured in **4 days**

Patient **Samiullah Shaikh** from *Mumbai* age **72 yrs** reported to N.I.C.E with the symptoms of **Sore throat, Tiredness** on **24-Jun-20** with comorbidities like **Hypertension , diabetes** got cured in **4 days**

Patient **Pushpalata Rao** from *Kalyan* age **51 yrs** reported to N.I.C.E with the symptoms of **Fever, Dry Cough, Headache, Body ache/muscle ache, Tiredness** on **26-Jun-20** with comorbidity like **Hypertension** got cured in **7 days** under the N.I.C.E Care of **Ajit Kumar Burnwal**

Patient **Parveen Sultana** from *Hyderabad* age **58 yrs** reported to N.I.C.E with the symptoms of **Fever, Sore throat, Headache, Body ache/muscle ache, Tiredness** on **28-Jun-20** with comorbidity like **Hypertension** got cured in **7 days** under the N.I.C.E Care of **Kumar Shivam**

Patient **Meena Ramrakhyani** from *Ahmedabad* age **52 yrs** reported to N.I.C.E with the symptoms of **Headache, Body ache/muscle ache, Breathing difficulty** on **29-Jun-20** with comorbidity like **Low Blood Pressure** got cured in **4 days** under the N.I.C.E Care of **Meena Gupta**

N.I.C.E Practitioners

Here is the partial list of N.I.C.E. practitioners, who have been working day & night to help Covid-19/Influenza/ILI patients recover from the illness. Most of them are certified medical nutritionist from Lincoln University College, Malaysia.

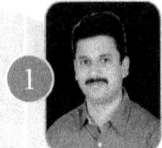

1

Name : Dr Nilesh Patil
Age : 45   **Place :** Jalgaon
Profession: MBBS-Ortho

2

Name : Dr Pallavi Patil
Age : 42   **Place :** Jalgaon
Profession: MBBS DMRE

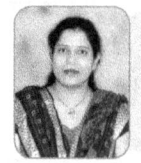

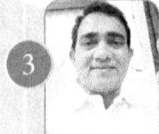

3

Name : Dr K B Tumane
Age : 59   **Place :** Nagpur
Profession: Chest Physician - Ex Chief Doctor (Deputy Director health services) of Nagpur Municipal corporation

4

Name : DGP Harinarayan Chari Mishra
Age : 43   **Place :** Indore
Profession: IPS Officer

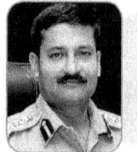

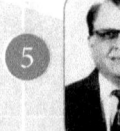

5

Name : Yogeshh Mittal
Age : 54   **Place :** Faridabad
Profession: Business

6

Name : Ashutosh Mittal
Age : 42   **Place :** Faridabad
Profession: Chairman of Scientific Instruments company

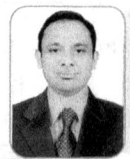

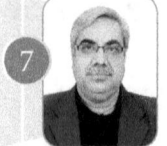

7

Name : Mahesh Kaushik
Age : 58   **Place :** Faridabad
Profession: Naturopathy Practitioner

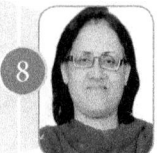

Name : Nirmala Pandey
Age : 58 **Place :** Gurugram
Profession: Software Testing Trainer and
practicing Naturopath

Name : Amrut Tikamchand Singhavi
Age : 42 **Place :** Amravati
Profession: Diabetes Educator

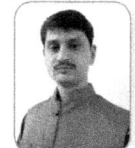

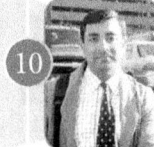

Name : Anurag Mittal
Age : 49 **Place :** Delhi
Profession: Govt Service

Name : Ananta Kumar Panda
Age : 44 **Place :** Gunupur
Profession: Business

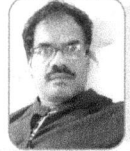

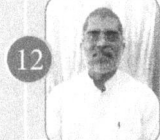

Name : Dr. Atul Ramesh Narkhede
Age : 48 **Place :** Surat
Profession: Homeopath

Name : Arvind Kumar Plaha
Age : 46 **Place :** Ludhiana
Profession: Yoga Teacher and Diabetes Educator

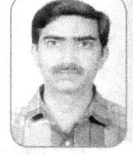

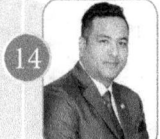

Name : Adarsha Narayan Pradhan
Age : 35 **Place :** Kathmandu
Profession: Psychologist/ Code-Blue Trainer/
Diabetes Educator

Name : Amit shimpi
Age : 33 **Place :** Nasik
Profession: Doctor

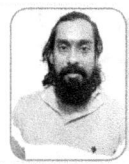

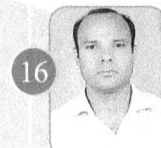

Name : Arun Kumar
Age : 40 **Place** : Bijnor
Profession: Teacher

16

Name : Ayan Halder
Age : 25 **Place** : Dankuni
Profession: Certified Diabetes Educator IVMB

17

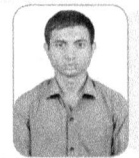

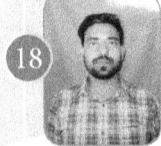

Name : Ajit Kumar Burnwal
Age : 30 **Place** : Pandaveswar
Profession: Operations Manager

18

Name : Ajeet Singh Foujdar
Age : 34 **Place** : Bharatpur
Profession: Indian Railways

19

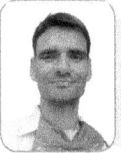

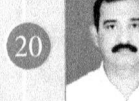

Name : Atul Jain
Age : 49 **Place** : New Delhi
Profession: Naturopath & Diabetic Educator

20

Name : Amit Aneja
Age : 36 **Place** : Panipat
Profession: Business man

21

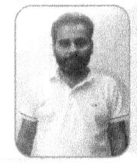

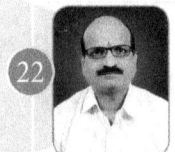

Name : Avinash Popatrao Sabare
Age : 51 **Place** : Ahmednagar
Profession: Agriculture Engineer and Mutual Fund Broker

22

Name : Ashish Agrawal
Age : 37 **Place** : Pune
Profession: Badminton Coach & Business

23

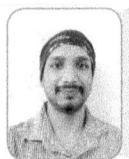

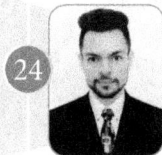

Name : Aggam
Age : 24 **Place :** Sydney
Profession: Health Nutritionist and Exercise
Professional

24

Name : Dr Akhilesh Sahu
Age : 35 **Place :** Raipur
Profession: Doctor (MPT,MS), PhD (Nature
Science & Medicine)

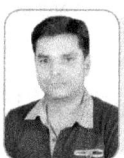

25

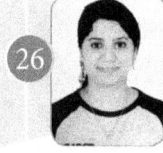
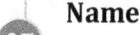

Name : Arpana Madhu Suvarna
Age : 38 **Place :** Thane
Profession: Service

26

Name : Alisha Massey
Age : 44 **Place :** Chandigarh
Profession: Certified Diabetes Educator

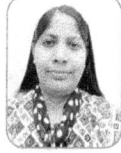

27

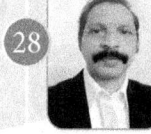

Name : Dr ABMK Vara Prasad
Age : 38 **Place :** Visakhapatnam
Profession: Doctor

28

Name : Brajakishore Sinha
Age : 28 **Place :** Silchar
Profession: Armed Forces

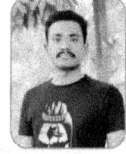

29

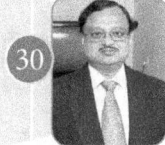

Name : Dr. Barin Kumar Roy
Age : 50 **Place :** Kolkata
Profession: Service (Teaching Profession) &
Diabetes Educator

30

Name : Bhupendra Singh Panwar
Age : 49 **Place :** Haridwar
Profession: Business

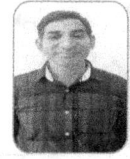

31

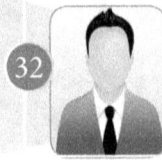

Name : Dr. Bhavani Vedicherla
Age : 41 **Place** : Hyderabad
Profession: Associate Scientist

32

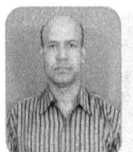

Name : Bimal Pal
Age : 41 **Place** : Bardhaman
Profession: Business

33

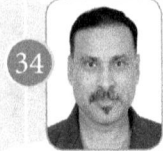

Name : Brijmohan Yadav
Age : 46 **Place** : Chennai
Profession: Professional Diabetes Educator

34

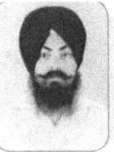

Name : Baltej Singh
Age : 35 **Place** : Barnala
Profession: Teacher

35

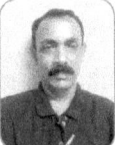

Name : Biswajit Datta
Age : 52 **Place** : Kanchanbari
Profession: Govt. Teacher

36

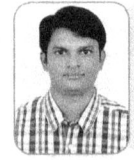

Name : B.Narendran
Age : 41 **Place** : Chennai
Profession: Diabetes Educator, Health Coach,
Electro Homeo Practitioner

37

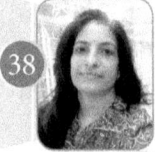

Name : Chitra Jain
Age : 50 **Place** : Pune
Profession: Yoga Instructor

38

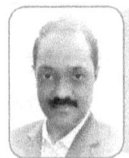

Name : Dr. C Rajasekhar
Age : 46 **Place** : Bengaluru
Profession: Health Coach

39

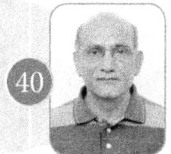

Name : Chotalia Sureshchandra
Age : 65 **Place :** Rajkot
Profession: Naturopath

40

Name : Chandramouli Kommanabilli
Age : 32 **Place :** Vizianagaram
Profession: Nutrition & Health Educator

41

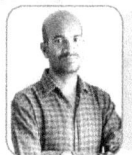

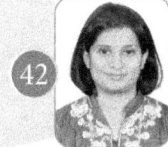

Name : Deepti V Helgaonkar
Age : 42 **Place :** Mumbai
Profession: Working with NABARD as Assistant
General Manager

42

Name : Dharmendra Kumar Pandey
Age : 40 **Place :** Delhi
Profession: Software Engineer

43

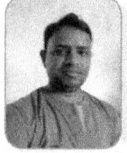

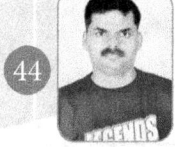

Name : Dushyant Chaturvedi
Age : 49 **Place :** Bharuch
Profession: Sr. manager / Financial Advisor

44

Name : Dilbag Singh
Age : 27 **Place :** Kotla Heran
Profession: Self Employed

45

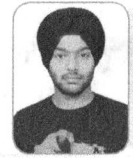

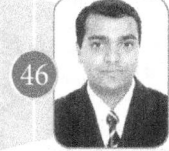

Name : Daniyal
Age : 38 **Place :** Dubai
Profession: BE

46

Name : Emandi Kumar Rao
Age : 40 **Place :** Jamshedpur
Profession: Sailor

47

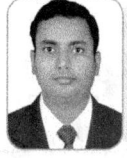

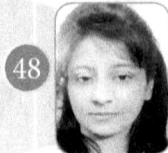

Name : Ekta Singh
Age : 36 **Place** : Lucknow
Profession: Self Employed

Name : Dr. Ekta Agarwal
Age : 44 **Place** : Kota
Profession: Diabetes Educator, (PhD Medicinal
Chemistry

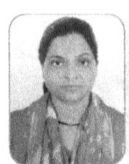

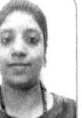

Name : Filda Don
Age : 32 **Place** : Aurangabad
Profession: Nurse

Name : Goma Ram
Age : 33 **Place** : Barmer
Profession: Private Job

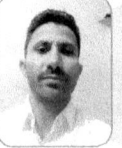

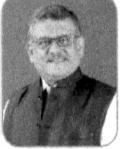

Name : Girish Banvi
Age : 55 **Place** : Dharwad
Profession: Wellness coach

Name : Gopinath Narayanam
Age : 62 **Place** : Hyderabad
Profession: Diabetes Educator, Yoga Therapist,
Medical Nutritionist

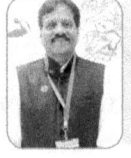

Name : Gaurav Jain
Age : 40 **Place** : Delhi
Profession: Aerospace and Aviation

Name : Dr Goutam Paul
Age : 47 **Place** : Kolkata
Profession: Doctor, DBMS

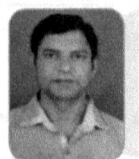

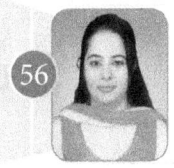

Name : Geetika Kapoor
Age : 32 **Place :** Faizabad, Ayodhaya
Profession: Nutritionist & Dietitian

56

Name : Dr Harsha Bhorhari
Age : 43 **Place :** Ahmedabad
Profession: Holistic Physician & Ayurvedic Consultant

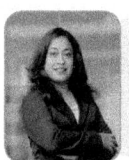

57

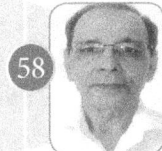

Name : Hulash Chand Sankhla
Age : 72 **Place :** Secunderabad
Profession: Ayurveda Practitioner

58

Name : Hemraj Jagannath Saner
Age : 46 **Place :** Mumbai
Profession: IT Project Manager , Certified Diabetes Educator

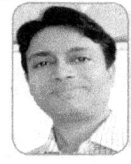

59

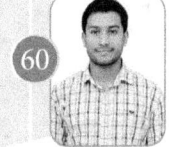

Name : Harshit Maheshwari
Age : 24 **Place :** New Delhi
Profession: Clinical Nutritionist

60

Name : Ishank Kumar Varshney
Age : 36 **Place :** Hathras
Profession: Teacher

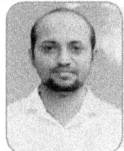

61

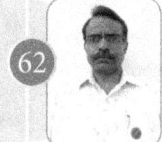

Name : Jitendra Ramaiya
Age : 48 **Place :** Gwalior
Profession: Computer Hardware Professional

62

Name : Jitendra Kumar Choubey
Age : 37 **Place :** Chapra, Saran
Profession: Diabetes Educator

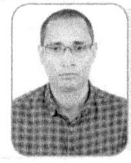

63

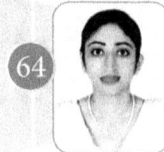

64

Name   : Jasmeet Kaur
Age   : 38   **Place :** New Delhi
Profession: Home Maker

65

Name   : Kumar Shivam
Age   : 21   **Place :** Pune
Profession: Student

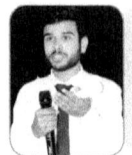

66

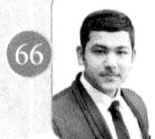

Name   : Kanishk Amarpuri
Age   : 21   **Place :** New Delhi
Profession: Yoga Teacher

67

Name   : Kamlakshi Shahdeo
Age   : 51   **Place :** Greensboro/USA
Profession: Homemaker, former Pharmaceutical
               Research Scientist

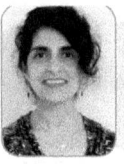

68

 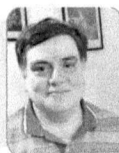

Name   : Kodur Venkata Ramana Sastry
Age   : 65   **Place :** Mumbai
Profession: Retired Associate Professor of
               Commerce

69

Name   : Dr. Kishan Pareek
Age   : 25   **Place :** Hyderabad
Profession: Public Health Student

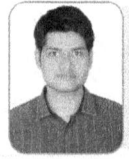

70

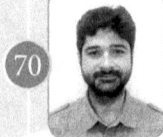

Name   : Kamal Dhawan
Age   : 36   **Place :** Ludhiana
Profession: Engineer/Businessman

71

Name   : Kapil Dev Sharma
Age   : 33   **Place :** Kalayat
Profession: Medical Nutritionist/ Diabetes
               Educator/ Code Blue Trainer

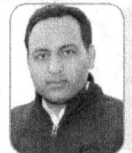

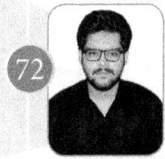

Name : Kunwar Aryaman
Age : 20 **Place :** Deoband
Profession: BHMS Final Year Student

Name : Kimti Lal
Age : 37 **Place :** Banga
Profession: Contractor

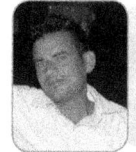

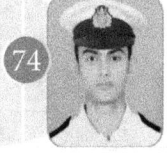

Name : Karan Shetty
Age : 27 **Place :** Mumbai
Profession: Marine Engineer

Name : Dr Karnraj Sandip Deshmukh
Age : 27 **Place :** Koregaon
Profession: Doctor

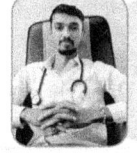

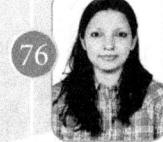

Name : Kavitha Gandhi
Age : 37 **Place :** Chennai
Profession: Home maker

Name : Lomash Anand
Age : 68 **Place :** Mahasamund
Profession: Training Instructor at LED.Plasma.
 Tv.Training institute

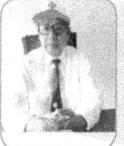

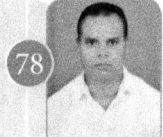

Name : Dr. Madan Lal
Age : 40 **Place :** Ambedkar Nagar
Profession: Naturopathy Doctor

Name : Dr. Manoj Kumar Sharma
Age : 33 **Place :** Chandauli
Profession: BHMS

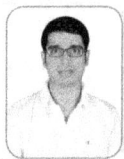

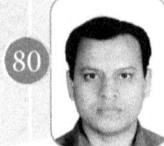

Name : Manjunath BV
Age : 37 **Place :** Bengaluru
Profession: Deputy Manager Finance

Name : Manish Arya
Age : 28 **Place :** Gurugram
Profession: Yoga Trainer

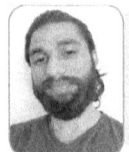

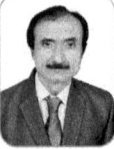

Name : Madhuri Anand Kinikar
Age : 48 **Place :** Mumbai
Profession: Naturopathy Practitioner

Name : Milesh D. Sahare
Age : 30 **Place :** Mumbai
Profession: Teacher

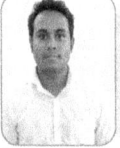

Name : Mushtaque Ahmad
Age : 65 **Place :** Siwan
Profession: Teacher

Name : Mohammad Rahil Nasim Ahmed Shaikh
Age : 21 **Place :** Mumbai
Profession: Optometrist

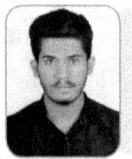

Name : Mansi Thaker
Age : 31 **Place :** Chennai
Profession: Food Safety Consultant

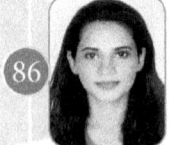

Name : Meena Gupta
Age : 57 **Place :** Kolkata
Profession: Dietitian, Diabetic Educator

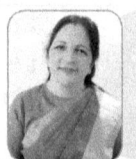

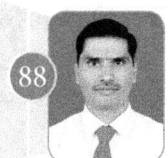

Name : Dr. Narasinhaswami Mamdyal
Age : 39 **Place :** Solapur
Profession: Ayurveda Practitioner & Neuro
Therapist

(88)

Name : Nishan Singh Jamwal
Age : 39 **Place :** Jammu
Profession: Assistant Accounts Officer

(89)

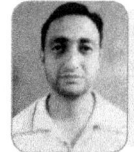

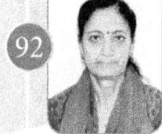

Name : Dr Nidhi Jain
Age : 42 **Place :** Mandleshwar
Profession: Homoeopath

(90)

Name : Nihar Ranjan Rout
Age : 52 **Place :** Bhubaneswar
Profession: Senior Business Associate in LIC of
India

(91)

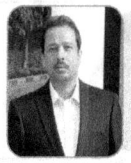

Name : Neelima Chatterjee
Age : 63 **Place :** New Delhi
Profession: Naturopath, Diabetes Educator

(92)

Name : Nilima Nitin Bhatkar
Age : 45 **Place :** Amravati
Profession: Sujok Therapist

(93)

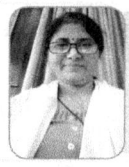

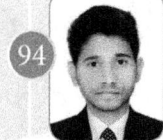

Name : Nishu Sandhya
Age : 23 **Place :** Janjgir Champa
Profession: Student/Singer

(94)

Name : Dr Pankaj Chaudhary
Age : 39 **Place :** Kanpur
Profession: BHMS

(95)

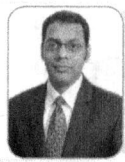

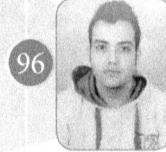

Name : Pratik Anand
Age : 31 **Place** : Delhi
Profession: Travel agency

96

Name : P. K. Sharma
Age : 46 **Place** : Ghaziabad
Profession: Teacher

97

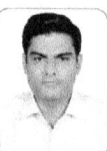

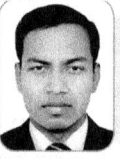

Name : Premkumar Krishnan
Age : 55 **Place** : Coimbatore
Profession: Business

98

Name : Prabin Nanda
Age : 35 **Place** : Bolangir
Profession: Diabetes Educator

99

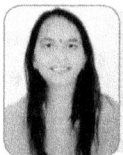

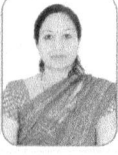

Name : Preethi Katariya
Age : 36 **Place** : Bengaluru
Profession: Naturopath

100

Name : Punyaapriya
Age : 26 **Place** : Delhi
Profession: Psychology Teacher

101

Name : Pragya Jha
Age : 39 **Place** : Indore
Profession: Diabetes Educator

102

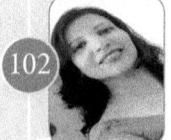

Name : Pradeep Chauhan
Age : 36 **Place** : Palghar
Profession: Healthcare

103

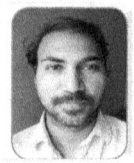

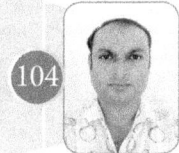

Name   : Dr Parmanand Patil
Age   : 34   **Place :** Jalgaon
Profession: BHMS

104

Name   : Dr Puran Sharma
Age   : 45   **Place :** New Delhi
Profession: Holistic Lifestyle Coach

105

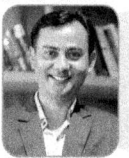

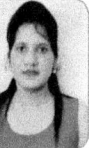

Name   : Prabhjot Kaur
Age   : 26   **Place :** Mohali
Profession: Doctor

106

Name   : Rupesh Kumar
Age   : 31   **Place :** Banka
Profession: Diabetes Educator, Advance Training
                     on Nutrition

107

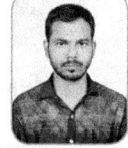

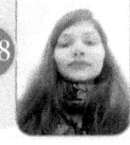

Name   : Rishu Garg
Age   : 33   **Place :** Panchkula
Profession: Lawyer and French Trainer

108

Name   : Rajendra Gorakharao Patil
Age   : 49   **Place :** Jalgaon
Profession: Business (electronic)

109

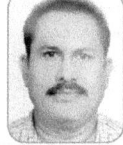

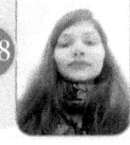

Name   : Rajwinder Kaur
Age   : 26   **Place :** Banga
Profession: Nursing

110

Name   : Ritesh Yadav
Age   : 23   **Place :** Ghazipur
Profession: Health Department

111

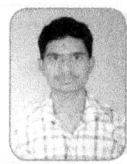

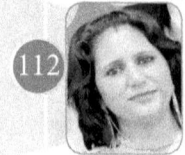

Name : Renu Garg
Age : 44   **Place :** Solan
Profession: Medical Nutritionist

Name : Dr. Reena Thakur
Age : 33   **Place :** Bonn
Profession: Dentist

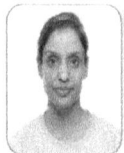

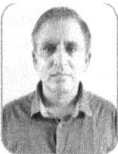

Name : Ravi Verma
Age : 62   **Place :** Raipur
Profession: Sr. Journalist

Name : Rahul Bansal
Age : 34   **Place :** Khandwa
Profession: Trading Business

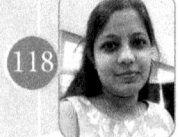

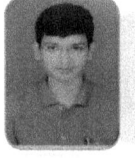

Name : Dr Rajendra Prasad Kumawat
Age : 53   **Place :** Jaipur
Profession: Sports Physiotherapist

Name : Rishabh Jain
Age : 60   **Place :** Delhi
Profession: Chemist

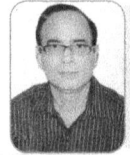

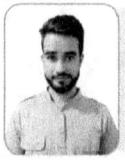

Name : Ruchi Surana
Age : 33   **Place :** Dubai
Profession: Reinsurance Analyst (Qualified Nutritionist)

Name : Raushan Kumar
Age : 25   **Place :** New Delhi
Profession: Floor Manager in an Ayurvedic Clinic

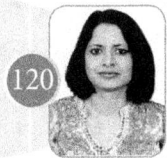

Name : Ritu Singh
Age : 46   **Place :** Agra
Profession: Nutritionist

Name : Raj Kishore Kodwani
Age : 52   **Place :** Bhopal
Profession: Acupressure Therapist

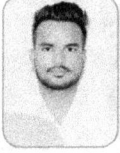

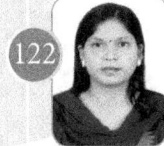

Name : Rekha Gupta
Age : 43   **Place :** New Delhi
Profession: Clinical Researcher

Name : Rajat Bharti
Age : 26   **Place :** Pathankot
Profession: Biotechnologist

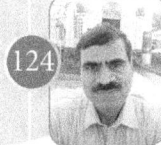

Name : Rajeev Kumar
Age : 52   **Place :** Agra
Profession: Engineer

Name : Ravinder Singh Kanwar
Age : 44   **Place :** Hoshiarpur
Profession: Acupressure / Acupuncture/
        Alternative Med. Practitioner

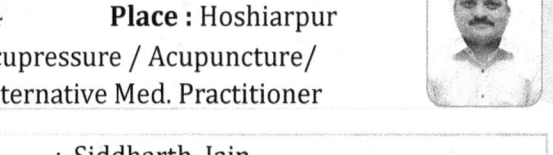

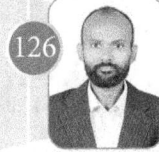

Name : Siddharth Jain
Age : 33   **Place :** Ghaziabad
Profession: Engineer

Name : Sayed Shah
Age : 32   **Place :** Mumbai
Profession: Student

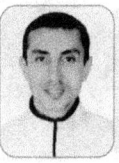

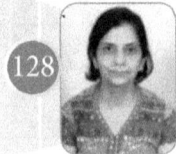

Name : Dr Seema Arora
Age : 53 **Place :** Una
Profession: Doctor

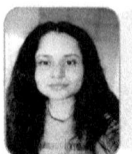

Name : Shubhangi Godse
Age : 25 **Place :** Pune
Profession: Software Engineer

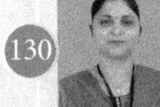

Name : Dr. Shikha Srivastava
Age : 41 **Place :** New Delhi
Profession: Assistant Professor

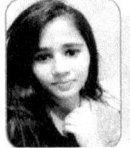

Name : Sheetal Kanwar
Age : 19 **Place :** Bhiwadi
Profession: Student

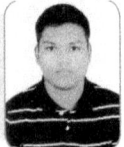

Name : Sourav Bysack
Age : 25 **Place :** Dankuni
Profession: Private Tutor

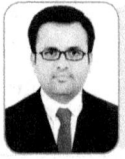

Name : Sanjay Dhaduk
Age : 37 **Place :** Bengaluru
Profession: Entrepreneur

Name : Sanjay Goopta
Age : 51 **Place :** New Delhi
Profession: Health Coach

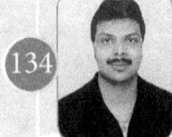

Name : Shikha Saxena
Age : 55 **Place :** Lucknow
Profession: Diabetes Educator

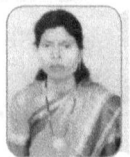

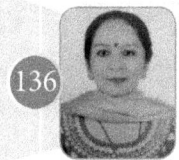

Name : Simi Handa
Age : 55 **Place :** New Delhi
Profession: Pharmacist

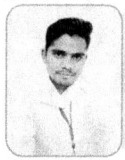

Name : Suresh Kumar Yadav
Age : 27 **Place :** Mandla
Profession: Neurotherapist

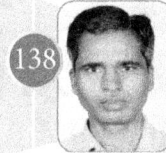

Name : Shiv Dular
Age : 52 **Place :** New Delhi
Profession: Code Blue Trainer

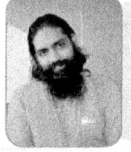

Name : Santosh Guruji
Age : 36 **Place :** Mumbai
Profession: Yog Guru

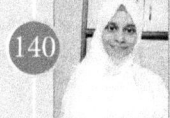

Name : Shaikh Iqra Ayaz
Age : 19 **Place :** Mumbai
Profession: BAMS Student

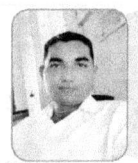

Name : Sudhir Kumar
Age : 39 **Place :** Rewari
Profession: Chemistry Lecturer

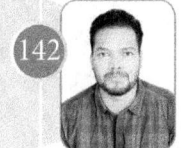

Name : Sraban Baraik
Age : 26 **Place :** Balangir
Profession: Independent Business Entrepreneur

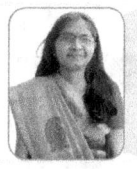

Name : Sushama Bengani
Age : 56 **Place :** Bengaluru
Profession: Qualified Naturopath

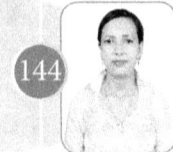

Name : Suman Chauhan
Age : 33 **Place :** Ambala
Profession: Doctor

Name : Samir Das
Age : 48 **Place :** New Delhi
Profession: Yoga Instructor

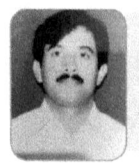

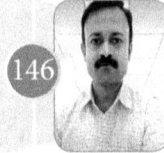

Name : Suresh Venkatrao Garad
Age : 42 **Place :** Latur
Profession: A Pharmacist, Health Educator ,
Naturopathy Practitioner

Name : Sounak Das
Age : 19 **Place :** Kharagpur
Profession: Medical Nutritionist

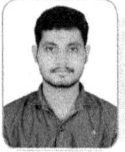

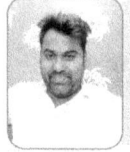

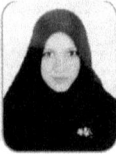

Name : Shaikh Warisha Nasim
Age : 19 **Place :** Mumbai
Profession: Student of BUMS Course

Name : Shahzada Alam
Age : 25 **Place :** Kolkata
Profession: Business

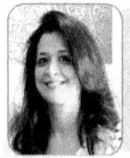

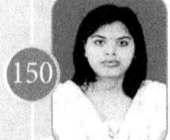

Name : Sashapra Chakrawarty
Age : 38 **Place :** Ranchi
Profession: Teaching

Name : Dr. Sunita Arya
Age : 53 **Place :** Hyderabad
Profession: Clinical Nutritionist (PhD. in
Nutrition)

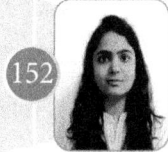

Name : Shreya Gadiya
Age : 25 **Place :** Udaipur
Profession: Yoga Teacher, Naturopathy and Acupressure Therapist

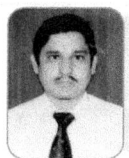

Name : Subhas Mukherjee
Age : 44 **Place :** Raniganj
Profession: Panchgavya Consultant

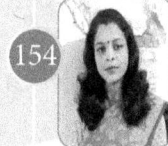

Name : Sneha Sinha
Age : 31 **Place :** Patna
Profession: Nurse

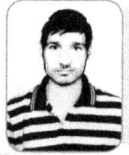

Name : Shashwat Kumar
Age : 26 **Place :** Patna
Profession: Health Practitioner

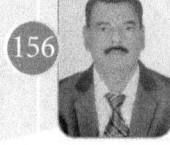

Name : Syed Wajid Husain
Age : 62 **Place :** Thane
Profession: Lawyer

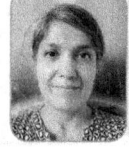

Name : Seema Manikkoth
Age : 51 **Place :** Mumbai
Profession: Service

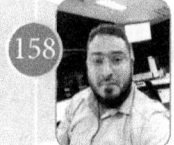

Name : Syed Babar Ahmed
Age : 39 **Place :** Hyderabad
Profession: EDI Specialist

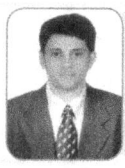

Name : Satish Kumar Varma Vuppalapati
Age : 39 **Place :** Hyderabad
Profession: Network Architect

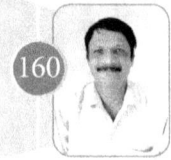

Name : Tapan Kumar Mahapatra
Age : 49 **Place :** Purba Medinipur
Profession: Computer System Administrator

Name : Thokchom Rameshwar Singh
Age : 42 **Place :** Imphal
Profession: Health Coach

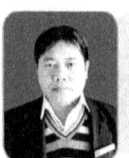

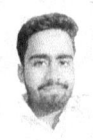

Name : Tahera Khaledi
Age : 29 **Place :** Hyderabad
Profession: Physiotherapist

Name : Utpal Roy
Age : 57 **Place :** North 24 Parganas
Profession: Business

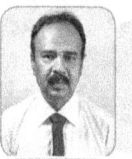

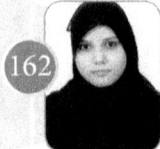

Name : Dr. Vishwajeet Khaiwal
Age : 23 **Place :** Shamli
Profession: BAMS

Name : Vasudev Roy
Age : 21 **Place :** Delhi
Profession: Health Consultant

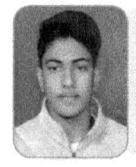

Name : Vinod Kumar Katheria
Age : 56 **Place :** New Delhi
Profession: Ayurvedic Physician

Name : Dr Vishal Singh Chauhan
Age : 40 **Place :** Greater Noida
Profession: BHMS, M.D

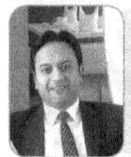

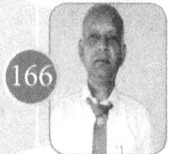

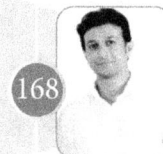

Name : Atish R Jaiswal
Age : 34   **Place :** Pune
Profession: Medical nutritionist Harvard/ Diabetes
Educator IVMB

Name : Bhagwan Dass
Age : 60   **Place :** Unnao
Profession: Health Adviser

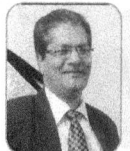

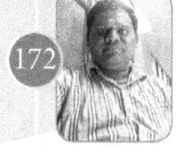

Name : Ranjan Ghosh
Age : 49   **Place :** Bhadrakali, Uttarpara
Profession: Health Worker

Name : Dr. Sanjay Kumar Patel
Age : 49   **Place :** RaeBareli
Profession: Homoeopathic Physician

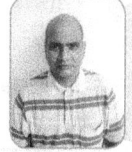

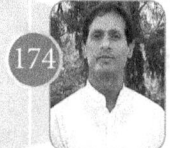

Name : Sameer Pandit
Age : 39   **Place :** Raigarh
Profession: Self Employed

Name : Manish
Age : 36   **Place :** Delhi
Profession: Engineer

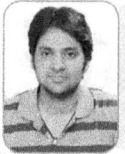

Name : Narendra Singh Pate
Age : 48   **Place :** Bhilai
Profession: Employee (Bhilai Steel Plant, SAIL) &
Business

Name : Kiran Jeet Kaur
Age : 38   **Place :** Chandigarh
Profession: Self employed (deals in organic
farming and food production)

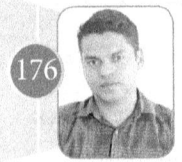

Name : Amitkumar Ramdas Naik
Age : 40 **Place :** Ponda
Profession: Health Coach

176

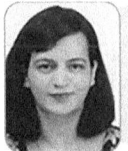

Name : Sandra Fernandes Paes
Age : 42 **Place :** Salmiya
Profession: Service

177

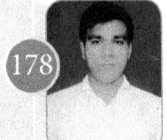

Name : Sanjay Sah
Age : 26 **Place :** Arrah
Profession: Homeopath

178

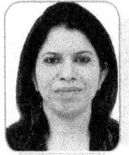

Name : Hema Singh
179 **Age** : 50 **Place :** Delhi
Profession: Diabetes Educator

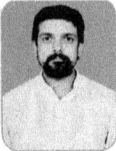

Name : Prakrit Kumar Singh
Age : 27 **Place :** Ranchi
Profession: Karate Instructor

180

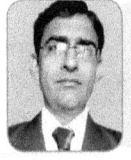

Name : Dharmendra Kumar Singh
181 **Age** : 42 **Place :** Patna
Profession: Diabetes Educator

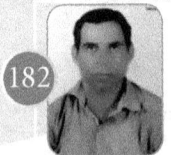

Name : Naveen Bhatia
Age : 56 **Place :** Bengaluru
Profession: Diabetes Educator

182

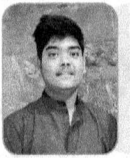

Name : Dr Tushar Bansal
183 **Age** : 22 **Place :** Khariar Road
Profession: Diabetes Educator, Medical Nutritionist

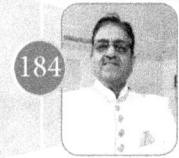

Name : Vijay Wadagbalkar
Age : 63 **Place :** Mumbai
Profession: Diabetes Educator

Name : Vineet Khaitan
Age : 36 **Place :** Kolkata
Profession: Assistant Office and Trading Operation

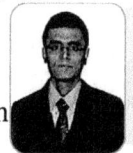

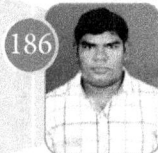

Name : Bala Showry Rudrapogu
Age : 39 **Place :** Amravathi
Profession: Catholic Priest & Lawyer

Name : Dr. Hemant Bafana
Age : 50 **Place :** Pune
Profession: Naturopath

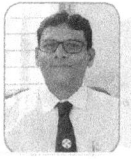

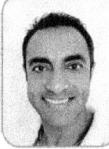

Name : Vikrant Singh Dogra
Age : 43 **Place :** Sydney
Profession: Certified Diabetes Educator

Name : Rajesh Tiwari
Age : 48 **Place :** Jabalpur
Profession: Railway Protection Force

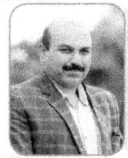

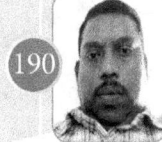

Name : Chandrashekhar Palikondawar
Age : 56 **Place :** Pusad
Profession: Diabetes Educator

Name : Masood Ahmad Khan
Age : 62 **Place :** Gujranwala
Profession: Certified Diabetes Educator

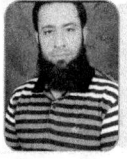

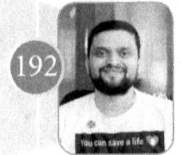

Name : Dr. Rakesh J Dashpute
Age : 40 **Place :** Bengaluru
Profession: Certified Diabetes Educator

(192)

Name : Sripada Kumar Baidya
Age : 47 **Place :** Kolkata
Profession: Ayurvedic Consultant

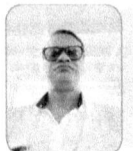

(193)

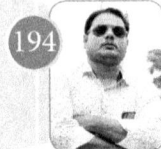

Name : Ajay Singh
Age : 39 **Place :** Sitapur
Profession: Ayurvedic Consultant

(194)

Name : Bibhuti Barik
Age : 33 **Place :** Bolangir
Profession: Medical Representative

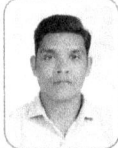

(195)

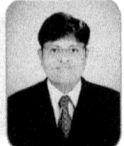

Name : Vivek Subhash Tarate
Age : 30 **Place :** Satara
Profession: Pharmacist, Code Blue Trainer,
Certified Diabetes Educator

(196)

Name : Nitin Jain
Age : 34 **Place :** Kishangarh
Profession: Software Developer, Diabetes Educator

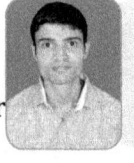

(197)

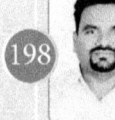

Name : Vishal Bekellu
Age : 36 **Place :** Pune
Profession: Owner of Review Company, Diabetes
Educator

(198)

Name : Mrs Kavita Jain
Age : 56 **Place :** Kochi
Profession: Diabetes Educator

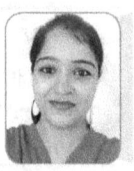

(199)

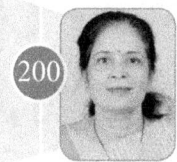

Name : Meena Joshi
Age : 50 **Place :** Gujarat
Profession: Teacher, Diabetes Educator

Name : Shivaji Balu Kulal
Age : 32 **Place :** Pune
Profession: Naturapath , Yoga Trainer, Diabetes Educator

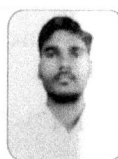

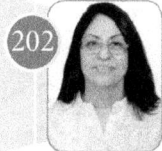

Name : Nanu Gadhok
Age : 65 **Place :** Mohali
Profession: Self Employed and Training Institute

Name : Mehershobha P Vyas
Age : 50 **Place :** Surat
Profession: Homeopath, Diabetes Educator

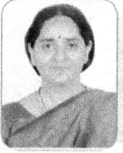

Name : Ajay Pal Singh
Age : 60 **Place :** Faridabad
Profession: Nathropath, Alternative Medicine Practitioner

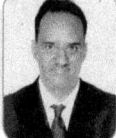

Name : Balasubramanium S
Age : 42 **Place :** Mumbai
Profession: Yoga Trainer, Diabetes Educator

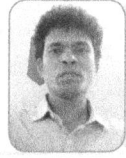

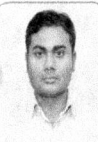

Name : Pankaj Kumar
Age : 24 **Place :** Kanpur Nagar
Profession: Self Employed, Diabetes Educator

Name : Dr. Syed Arif
Age : 45 **Place :** Kalaburagi
Profession: Medical Practitioner and University Lecturer

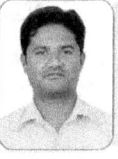

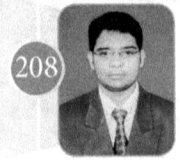

Name : Dr Madhab Nayak
Age : 32 **Place :** Berhampur
Profession: MBBS/MD, Diabetes Educator

Name : Mohana Ramaswamy
Age : 42 **Place :** London
Profession: Diabetes Educator

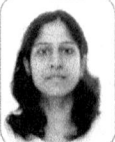

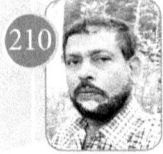

Name : Gobinda Lal Sarkar
Age : 62 **Place :** Habra
Profession: Retired from Accounts Department,
Medical Nutritionist

Name : Rajani Engu
Age : 31 **Place :** Hyderabad
Profession: MBBS/MD, Specialized In Gynaecology

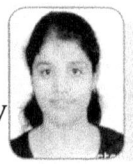

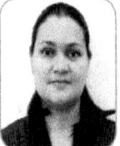

Name : Hameshel Kaur
Age : 39 **Place :** Pennsylvania
Profession: Diabetes Educator

Name : Rakesh Kumar Verma
Age : 61 **Place :** Rishikesh
Profession: Retired Military Engineer

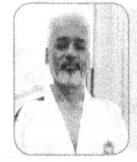

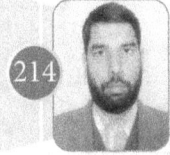

Name : Mohammad Firoz Alam
Age : 47 **Place :** Noida
Profession: Health Consultant/Software Engineer

Name : Mohammed Saleem
Age : 52 **Place :** Sharjah
Profession: Planning Manager - Industrial
Engineer

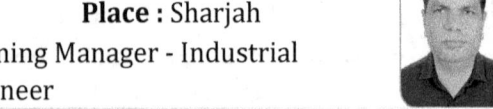

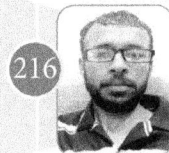

Name : Vijay Anand
Age : 32 **Place :** Mahasamund
Profession: Electronics Business/ Medical
Nutritionist

216

Name : Nilesh Talele
Age : 45 **Place :** Mumbai
Profession: IT Department, Naturopath

217

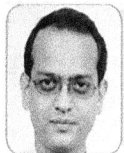

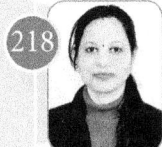

Name : Anjali Arya Chopra
Age : 46 **Place :** Vrindavan
Profession: Diabetes Educator, B.N.Y.H

218

Name : Sanjeev Kumar
Age : 47 **Place :** Patna
Profession: Internet Marketing

220

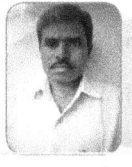

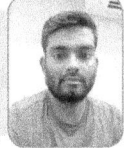

Name : Arun Kumar Upadhyay
Age : 33 **Place :** Howrah
Profession: Fitness Trainer and Diabetes
Educator

221

Name : Dr. Rajat Bharti
Age : 25 **Place :** Pathankot
Profession: Biotechnologist, Diabetes Educator,
RICH Course

222

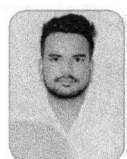

How to End Covid-19 Pandemic?

To know the answer to the above question, we need to go back to the first death allegedly due to Covid -19. It occurred on Jan 9, 2020, when a 61 year old patient died in Wuhan[49].

Two important factors need to be considered here:

1) The patient was already suffering from abdomen Cancer and liver disease, besides being old (61 yrs)[50].

2) No biopsy matter was taken after death[51].

With the above factors in consideration, how can one conclude that the death is due to SARS-CoV-2 and not due to Cancer or liver disease?

In fact, whenever autopsies were done on the dead bodies of supposedly Covid-19 patients[52], virus was never found to be the cause of death. For me, raising a doubt about SARS-CoV-2 to be the true cause of illness becomes more firm when I see the inconsistency in the 2nd RT –PCR Test diagnostic reports of my N.I.C.E patients .

The major inconsistencies are :

1) Patients still demonstrating symptoms of Flu, however, got the 2nd PCR test for Covid-19 to be negative (the first one was positive).

2) With many of the patients, showing 2nd RT–PCR Test for Covid-19 positive even after resolving all the symptoms (the first Covid-19 test was positive for all of them).

To put an end to the dispute, whether a particular pathogen is responsible for a disease, a gold standard test, called Koch's Postulate, was taken into consideration. It has been in use since 1890s and is relevant even today.

Even the SARS (2003) Corona virus fulfilled the Koch's Postulate[53] and hence established as a true cause of Severe Acute Respiratory Syndrome. However, in case of SARS-CoV-2, it had not been tested for Koch's Postulate[54]

Koch's Postulates[55]

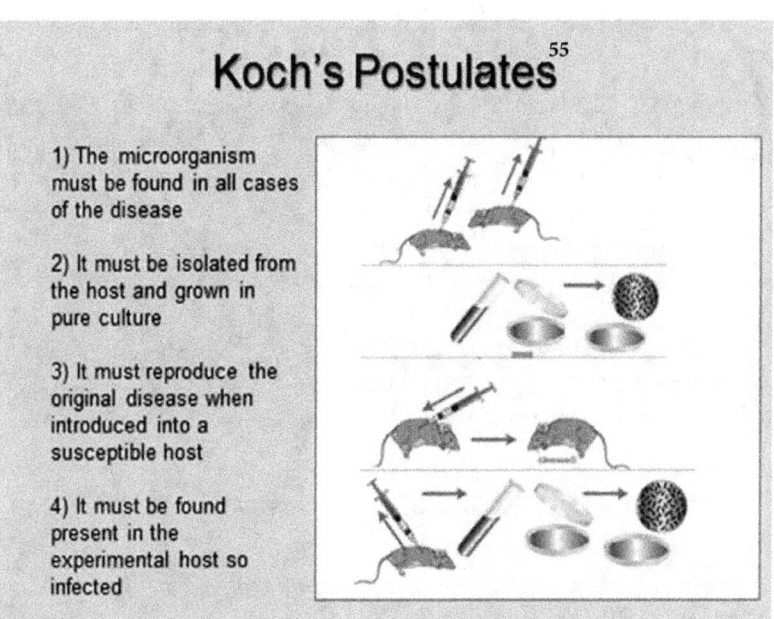

1) The microorganism must be found in all cases of the disease

2) It must be isolated from the host and grown in pure culture

3) It must reproduce the original disease when introduced into a susceptible host

4) It must be found present in the experimental host so infected

My conclusion and demand from regulating authorities are as follows:

1) Autopsy should be done on the suspected Covid-19 death before announcing it to be a Covid-19 death.

2) Koch's postulates should be fulfilled for SARS-CoV-2 virus; only then epidemic/pandemic can be truly established.

3) All Flu cases (including Covid-19) should be treated with three step Flu diet, at home itself, as with this strategy, we have achieved 0% CFR and more than 80% recovered rate within 72 hours of three step Flu diet intervention.

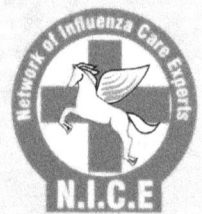
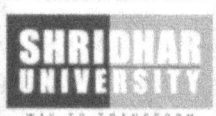

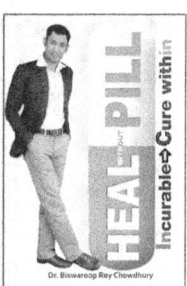
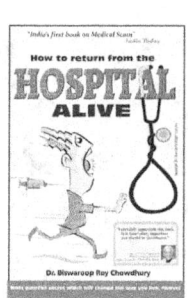
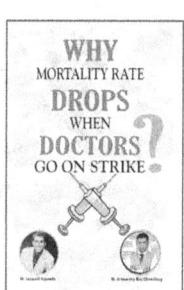
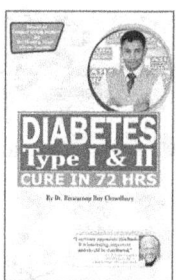
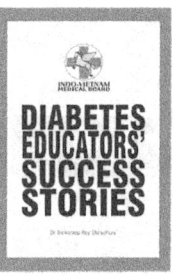
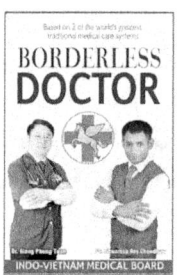
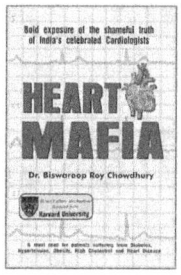
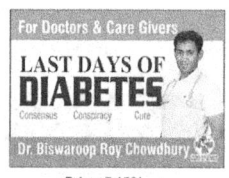
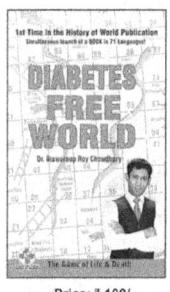
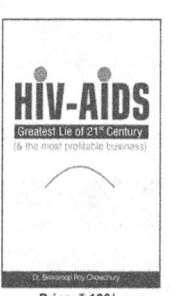
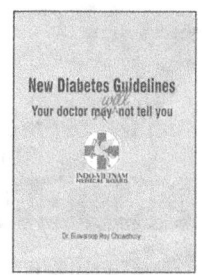
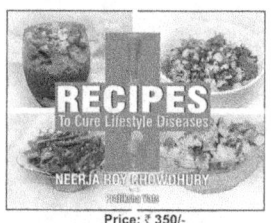

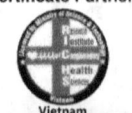

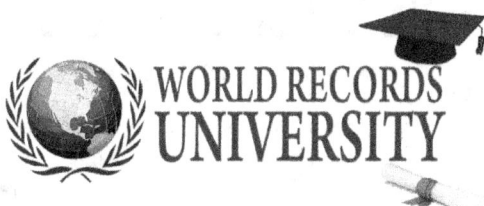

WORLD RECORDS UNIVERSITY

World Records University is an autonomous university formed by the conglomeration of National Record Books all across the globe. It has its registered office in UK, Vietnam and and India (Faridabad, Haryana).

World Records University has launched an Honorary Doctorate in Nature Science and Medicine in India with content based on Indo-Vietnam Medical Board.

Honorary Doctorate in Nature Science and Medicine:

Eligibility Criteria:

World Records University Invites applications for Honorary Doctorate from health practitioners practicing in the following fields:

- Allopathy
- Ayurveda
- Naturopathy
- Homeopathy
- Acupressure
- Acupuncture
- Physiotherapy
- Yoga
- Psychoneurobics
- Unani
- Chromotherapy
- Aromatherapy
- Magnet Therapy
- Reiki
- Neuro Linguistic Planning
- Osteopathy
- Pranic Healing
- Reflexology
- Siddha Medicine
- Qi

Steps to claim your Honorary Doctorate in Nature Science and Medicine:

Step 1: The applicant has to pass an online screening test(in Hindi, English, Vietnamese, Nepali) conducted by World Records University.

Step 2: You will be given an online study material.

Step 3: Submit doctorate application form (DAF) on the basis of your understanding of the study material (provided by World Records University).

Step 4: Write thesis on the basis of the format provided by World Records University.

Step 5: Submit your thesis.

Step 6: World Records University will authenticate the originality of your thesis and on acceptance by the panel of experts World Records University will confer you the Honorary Doctorate.

Step 7: Your thesis will be published in World Records University's annual publication.

For details contact us at www.worldrecordsuniversity.co.uk
E-mail: info@worldrecordsuniversity.com, Phone:+91-129-2510534, +91-9555008451

 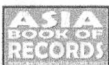 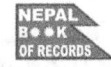

The Ultimate honor in alternative medicine...

Let every morning be the Hunza Morning

If you have decided to pick only one of my suggestions for the sake of your health, then take this suggestion:

Stop consuming tea specially, morning tea. The early morning tea makes the inner lining of your intestinal wall acidic, as after a long night of fasting your stomach is empty and craving for food. An acidic stomach on a regular basis is the single biggest cause of all kind of inflammatory and lifestyle diseases including arthritis, Diabetes etc.

How to stop craving of tea ⟶ Switch to Hunza Tea

Hunza Civilization: Hunza people are the Indians living at extreme northwest of India in Hindu Kush range. They are known to be one of the world's healthiest civilizations, often living up to the age of 110 years.

How to prepare Hunza Tea (serves four):

Ingredients:
- 12 Mint leaves(Pudina)
- 8 Basil Leaves(Tulsi)
- 4 Green cardamom (Elaichi)
- 2 gm Cinnamon (Dalchini)
- 20 gm Ginger (Adrak)
- 20 gm Jaggery (Gur)

Instructions:
- Take 4 cups of water in a tea pan
- Add all ingredients, simmer it for 10mins
- Add a dash of lemon juice and serve hot or cold

For those who are too lazy to collect the above ingredients (to make their own hunza tea) may order

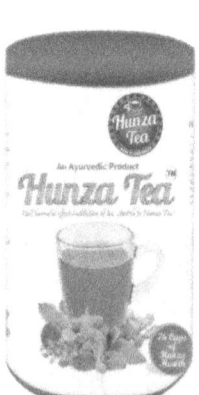

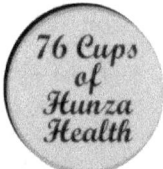

76 Cups of Hunza Health

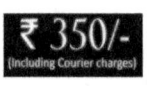

₹ 350/-
(Including Courier charges)

You may place your order at:

Dynamic Memory Pvt. Ltd.
B-121, 2nd Floor, Green Fields,
Faridabad (Haryana)
Mobile No.:+91-9312286540,
E-mail: biswaroop@biswaroop.com

Log on to www.biswaroop.com to buy products

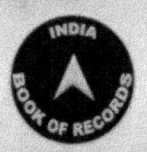
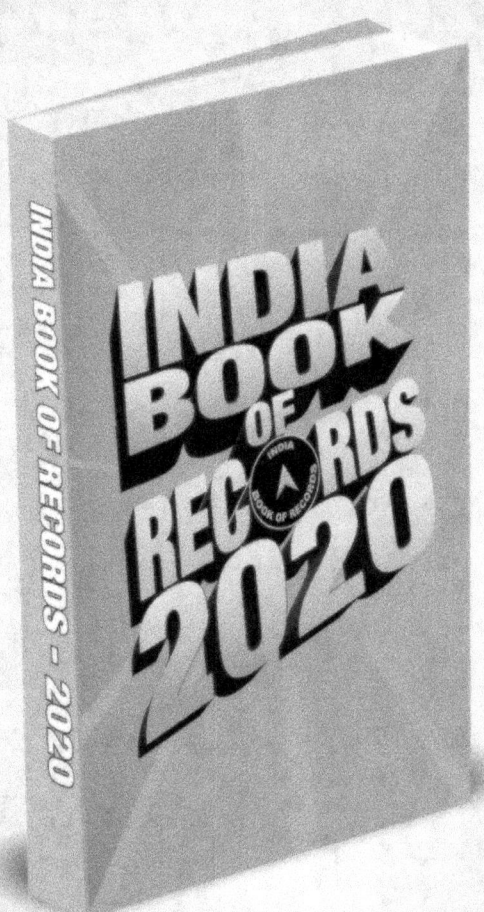
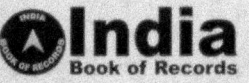

It's your chance to reverse Diabetes
Join

DIABETES
72hrs Program
3 Days Residential Tour

Be under the direct supervision of
internationally renowned medical nutritionist

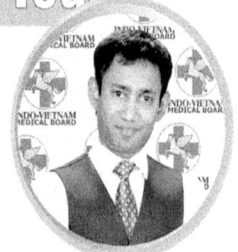

Dr. Biswaroop Roy Chowdhury
and his medical team for **3** days
**Free yourself from
the burden of 3 D's**

Diagnosis, Drugs and Diabetes
.....Forever

You can do it in 3 steps:

Step-1 : To Know about the program logon to www.biswaroop.com/residential-tour
Step-2: Book a seat at the above link or contact us at+91-9312286540 or mail at biswaroop@biswaroop.com
Step-3: Spend 3 life transforming days with us.

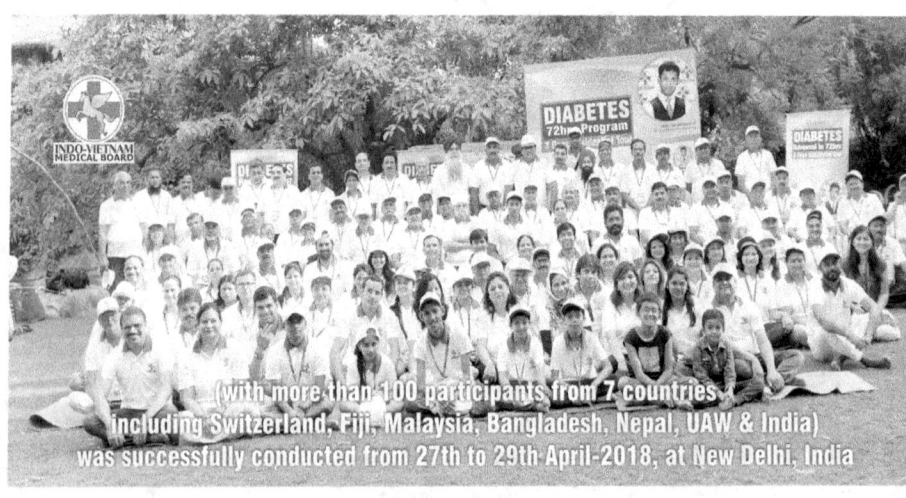

(with more than 100 participants from 7 countries
including Switzerland, Fiji, Malaysia, Bangladesh, Nepal, UAW & India)
was successfully conducted from 27th to 29th April-2018, at New Delhi, India

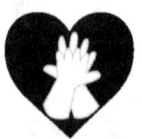 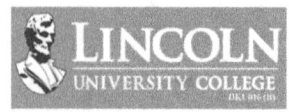 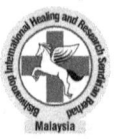

Code Blue Certification Training
(Protocol To Reverse And Manage Chest Pain, Heart Attack And Cardiac Arrest)

Overview: Aim of the training is to equip the clinicians and the layman with the skills to successfully manage and revive a chest pain, heart attack, and cardiac arrest victim. It is an evidence-based training with reference from more than 100 research papers (available in Pubmed) since the propagation of Cardiopulmonary Resuscitation, which started in the early 1960s.

Duration: One-month certification course

Content:
1) History of Cardiac Resuscitation
2) Diagnosing a cardiac arrest
3) Principle of Cardiac Resuscitation
4) Cardiac compression technique
5) Comparison of popular CPR Vs Cardiac Compression
6) Principle and practice of automated external defibrillator
7) The latest evidence base of the widespread practice of :
   a) Oxygen therapy
   b) Administering epinephrine
   c) Percutaneous coronary intervention (PCI)
   d) Bypass Surgery
8. 3 Step protocol to manage
   a) Chest Pain
   b) Heart Attack
   c) Cardiac Arrest (AED required)
9. Prevention of future chest pain/heart attack/ cardiac arrest
10. CME & practice to be a successful "Code Blue Trainer".

Training material:
1) Code Blue Trainer's Reference Book.
2) Cardiac compression training tool
3) Code Blue Trainer's practice T-shirt.

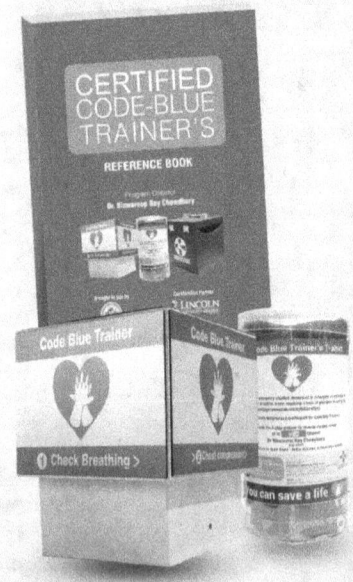

Course Fee:
INR 21,000/-
(including GST + Courier)

Mode of Training:
1) Training through online / video modules
2) Practice & evaluation through online/video conferencing

To register go to www.biswaroop.com/codebluetraining

CALL US :+91-9312286540 MAIL US: biswaroop@biswaroop.com